The Art of
Emotional Wisdom

Ute –
Thanks for sharing the journey.
There's no place like OM.
— Liam

The Art of
Emotional Wisdom

Liam Quirk

Unlimited Publishing
Bloomington, Indiana

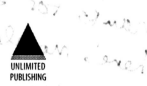

in wondrous gratitude to my teachers
for their guiding wisdom

Acknowledgments

I am grateful for and appreciate the many bright and creative people who have helped out on this multi-year project—reviewers, editors, readers and publishing pros, including Steve Bye, Jim Granger, Hank Beckhoff, Tracy Cunningham, Merlin Yockstick, Jean Haug, Shakaya, Buck, Donald Schnell, Shelley Milhous, Erin Defieux, Joe Yeager, Elizabeth Joyce, Jim Currie, Rob Ivker, Marilyn Diamond, Sherry Snow of SS Design, and Dan Snow of Unlimited Publishing. I am also very grateful for those who have contributed through their support of me and my work—clients, family, and friends. Thank you all.

Contents

Introduction

The fundamental assumption of this book is that we are all more than good enough to really be ourselves. We are smart enough, rich enough, and talented enough to be the best version of ourselves that we could ever imagine.

Where we fall short is that we don't really see ourselves. We don't see and experience the beauty of our being for who we are now, in this and every moment. One reason for this undersight is that for the most part we don't grasp the truth that all of our experiences have relentlessly shaped us and guided us to our greatest potentials for love and creativity—and continue to do so. We also generally don't fully understand that we are evolutionarily destined to be happy, and that our ignorance, especially our emotional ignorance, keeps us locked inside the seeds of our becoming.

What we would be wise to learn is that each of us carries within ourselves a gift, and this gift is the truth of our absolute worthiness, our most sacred divinity. Accepting this gift means that we will first of all have to unpack and transform the emotional woundedness it comes wrapped in. And we should know that this truth of our unconditional worthiness is a gift worth claiming, for there is a direct link between the emotional foundation of self-acceptance and the ability to create a life that satisfies our deepest yearnings for creative expression, true intimacy and authentic community.

The art of emotional wisdom means learning to recognize and understand our emotional woundedness so that it can be gracefully healed and our divinity revealed. Such healing is vitally important.

Our current confused fear and ignorance regarding emotion and emotional wounding has drastic and disastrous consequences for our well being, and the well being of our planet.

The good news is that the emotional healing that leads to emotional wisdom is not as difficult nor as heart-wrenching as we may fear. The aim of this book, therefore, is to be a sensible and practical guide for people who would like to make progress on the path of graceful emotional healing and fulfill their potentials for love and creativity.

In healing our emotional wounds we make room for the truth of our being to be more evident in our lives, which brings greater happiness and more heartfelt connection with others. My hope is that this book will offer you clear and easy-to-follow maps for unwinding the thoughts, energies and emotions that make up who you really are, so that your true colors, the unique rainbow of your being, can shine through to enrich your life and touch those you love.

The Highest Good of Happiness

Emotions make sense. This is true not only from the perspective that sees the causes and effects of emotional energies in our feelings and behavior, but also quite literally, as in: Emotions are a vital and inseparable part of the very foundation of our mind's sense-making. Whatever we think, feel, say or do, emotion is right there from the very beginning, a weave in the fabric of our being.

Often we are tempted to think that it is our minds or imaginations alone that have the upper hand or are even running the way we make sense of our world, and so we attempt to take an objective or emotion-free look at things to get a clearer picture. This, as it turns out, is a potentially tragic error, for such a habit limits our emotional engagement in the world, and therefore also our happiness. Alternately, we may project our fears or anger into everything we do, not realizing that this will only create more of the same. Emotion is a powerful creative force, and our disregard, fear and ignorance of emotion can only keep us from the happiness we most desire.

When it comes right down to it, our minds can no more function without emotion than our bodies can go without air. And when we learn to live on a low-emotion diet, we are zapping the zest for life that makes us want to get up in the morning. Even more, without a keen understanding and appreciation of emotion and its place in our overall human experience, we'll never learn to realize our potentials for love and creativity.

It may even be that our tendency to separate heart and head, or emotion and mind—whatever terms you use—is the result of our basic ignorance about the central role of emotion in all aspects of our thinking and well being. And living in a such a way—head disconnected from the heart—is ultimately not very satisfying, and certainly not fun. Nor beautiful. Yet joy, love and a sense of beauty—all emotionally rich—are our highest experiences, so right away we should understand that something is terribly wrong when we treat mind, one mode or aspect of experience, as if it were our highest, or our only, mode of experience. There is a much fuller picture, a much greater potential for human life than to live a life dominated or ruled by the mind.

Of course in reality there can be no real separation of the three modes of human experience—which will be referred to in this book as body, emotion, and mind—since they are all interconnected and interwoven with one another (a fact that turns out to be a very good thing, as we shall see). It is possible, however, and unfortunately all-too-prevalent in our culture to favor one of these modes at the expense of at least one of the others. It's like having a house with three magnificent picture windows that open out to different views, but getting stuck looking out just one of them while the others are draped shut.

This is not to say that we do not have built-in tendencies or predispositions for one of the modes, for we often do. Rather, what seems to happen is that we become experientially cut off from one or more of them. And when that happens, we are in serious trouble because all the aspects of our experience form one system, and doing without conscious connection to body, emotion or mind will drastically reduce our chances for the life of creative expression and joy that is our true potential.

This way of looking at our human experience, categorized into three overlapping and interconnected spheres or domains, is not new. In fact we are used to the now-standard holistic triad of body, mind and spirit as a way to understand the basic aspects or facets of our being. And such triads are commonly found throughout our spiritual traditions, including the Christian trinity of Father, Son and Holy Spirit. At the same time, we are also used to looking at our experience as a duality, either the classic body and mind duality, or the heart and head duality already mentioned—even when we then seek to overcome such dualistic thinking by referring to the bodymind or mind/body.

The triad of human experience I am introducing for the purposes of exploring the art of emotional wisdom, however, is somewhat different, for it takes the familiar body, mind and spirit triad and introduces emotion as one of the primary spheres, giving us body, emotion and mind. Actually, I generally prefer the term imagination to mind because *mind* has taken on a rather cold-hearted aspect due to our polarized, dualistic categorizations of body and mind or heart and head. For its familiarity, however, the term mind will be used throughout this book, though I will occasionally use imagination in contexts where the sense will be enriched by the associations of the word *imagination*.

And what of spirit? It is the basic assumption of the body, emotion and mind triad that spirit is infused throughout all aspects of our experience. Spirit, in other words, is not to be seen as something outside of our experience in any way. Body is infused with spirit as much as emotion or mind are infused with spirit, for spirit is our word for the creative intelligence and heartfelt knowingness underlying and supporting all of Creation. Having a separate category for spirit, from this perspective, is like trying to conceive of our world or universe without energy, when we know from physics that energy (in all its forms) is really all there is.

And the way we think about things really does matter. If we are conceiving of our experience in ways that actually limit that experience, and therefore also our potential for life's greatest experiences, then this is a serious matter. In fact the basic reason why we need to be consciously tuned in to all three aspects or modes of our experience is that all of our experiences form an overall design or system that is relentlessly working toward one goal: the realization of our potentials for love and creativity, and therefore our greatest happiness.

This is certainly a naïve or even foolish statement from the "real world" point of view that currently dominates our culture's beliefs about life, but perhaps the "realistic" view is another result of the basic misperceptions and faulty priorities regarding the human quest for fulfillment and happiness that are currently part of our world. Perhaps we are even caught in a loop of self-fulfilling prophecy— the standard "real world" belief system that will find justification for its fears and sense of limitation in the "reality" that system creates, thus reinforcing a flawed belief system. This, however, is getting a bit ahead of ourselves. What we need to do first is examine just how the three modes of our experience operate, and come to some understanding of why.

Becoming Fully Human

In the most basic sense, the fundamental insight of psychology, spirituality, religion—and indeed of all self-inquiry—is that we are always more than we consciously know ourselves to be. Science also appears to agree with the spirit of this point of departure, for science is quite comfortable with looking for and examining unseen forces like gravity that shape our world and therefore our conceptions of it. Perhaps in the final analysis, all fields of study are really just about mapping out and explaining just what it is that we don't yet know about who we are and where and how we live or could best live. This is equally true for the wisdom sciences, which at their best propose to integrate all of our acquired knowledge about what makes for a fulfilling life and give us a plan or road map.

And of course the reason we're looking for road maps in the first place is that we don't seem to be having enough of the kinds of experiences we most desire. In fact it wouldn't take too much for just about everyone to agree that moments of joyous clarity and transcendence are all-too-rare in our lives. Mostly we'd probably even settle for more moments of simple happiness than ask for the pie-in-the-sky mystical experiences of Oneness suggested by words like "joyous clarity" and "transcendence." After all, we've learned to keep our expectations low so that we can be pleasantly surprised rather than disappointed.

On the other hand, maybe we should be asking ourselves just why we're so sheepish. Don't we really want to believe that our experiences of joy represent the pure and true nature of existence, and that we can therefore find ways to increase those experiences? Isn't life truly the complete, awesome wonder we sometimes glimpse—even if we can't seem to keep our eyes open to that truth?

But since the more usual experiences of our lives convince us, by sheer percentage alone, that the joyous, transcendent happenings of life are the exception rather than the rule, we come up with all kinds of explanations for this state of affairs. Maybe, for example, we imagine ourselves to be involved in a cosmic battle of sorts where the forces of Good and Evil dictate how much joyous, loving experience will be made available. In darker times there will naturally be less bliss available than in lighter times—or we may even come to believe that what we know as human existence is the dark time, and a time after this life will be the time of light.

Yet no matter what we believe about the reasons for how much happiness and joy we experience on a daily basis—or whether we, as humans, even deserve such joy—our experience always comes down to the moment. Now, as the culmination of all human and personal history, is the only true experience we ever have. There is nothing but the ever-changing Right Now, try as we might to shake ourselves free of it, or try as we might to freeze the frame and hold on to an already fading moment.

From such a perspective, the statement from sages, saints and mystics that everything is already perfect makes perfect sense. That is because Now is always the only outcome of all that has come before, and now is the freshest, most real we can get—because in terms of our experience, it's really all there is.

This is not to say that the moment always feels good, or even that it should feel good or not good. The point is that the moment can only be what it is, and upon reflection this turns out to be more interesting and insightful than it may first appear—especially when we are concerned with understanding life so that we may make wise choices to make us happier.

From here it doesn't take much introspection to see that all of our activity is consciously and unconsciously based on this one aim: to create a life for ourselves that we find worth living, which means, at least theoretically, our happiest possible life. This is what Aristotle pointed out when he claimed that the highest good, the most worthy goal of human effort, is happiness, as shown by the fact that it is valued for its own sake and not as the means to something else.

So basically, our desire to understand life comes from, or is perhaps the same as, our desire to make choices that will make us happier. Of course happiness and joy also feel good, and we will have to look closely at this link between pleasure and humanity's highest good— as well as attempt to define what is meant by happiness in the first place. For now, however, it is enough to realize that regardless of how aware we are of it, the quest to understand life and to create happiness is at the heart of all of our thoughts and actions.

It is even possible to go as far as to say that making sense of our personal lives, and of life in general, is the primary activity of human existence. We may find it surprising to recognize that in the broadest view, making sense of things is indeed our only activity (if we include of course carrying out the conclusions we've come to). We do what we do in order to discover or satisfy what is right for us, all the way from ensuring our physical existence to contemplating the nature of that existence—and everything in-between. Making sense is the key phrase here, which for now we can think of as getting things as close as we possibly can to the point that they feel or seem good and right (which means approaching what makes us happy). And that is basically what we are all up to, all of the time.

Due to this sole human activity of making sense of our personal lives and the lives of others, we have, over the ages, accumulated a wealth of knowledge, material goods and institutions—all of it providing in some fashion an answer or answers to satisfy our desire to make sense of things so that we can be as happy as possible. Or another way to phrase the same idea is to say that humans have developed ways to provide satisfying answers to the question of what human life is all about. This is an equivalent statement because the desire to make sense of things, to get as close as possible to the point where things feel or seem right, can also be understood as the question: What is life?

This may seem like an almost ridiculously reduced explanation of life, but it is important to take the largest, simplest view if we want to see how we can go about trying to understand something as complex as life while we are positioned seemingly in the middle of it. And what we really need to see at this point is that each individual born into human life continues in the human tradition of trying to make sense of it all—with the help and hindrance of all these accumulated answers, which are consciously and, as it turns out, unconsciously passed down through the forms of human meaning, most notably behavior, language and culture.

Even at this general level of discussion there are already some rather interesting and revealing conclusions to be drawn. First of all, the activity of making sense of our lives assumes that our lives can indeed make sense, that there is in fact an order, design or meaning to life that seems to be about being as happy as possible. But even if we were to take this meaning to be simple physical survival, we have to allow for the existence of a system or design that supports this survival (such as the ecosystem).

Another interesting and important assumption we need to make is that we have memory. We can remember and compare moments, things, ideas, and then from those memories we can begin to choose (for example on the physical level, being warm versus being cold) what makes more sense. Also, as humans we have the ability to imagine what we have never before experienced, and this faculty of imagination lies at the heart of our sense-making activity because it creates a multitude of possibilities, of choices. Of course equally important at this point are our emotional and physical evaluations of each moment of experience, for our evaluations concerning the quality of each experience or imagined experience are what inform our decisions to seek out, re-create or avoid particular experiences.

In essence, therefore, all humans are seekers. Our sense-making stems from the desire to be able to arrange things so that they seem and feel good and right—which naturally makes us happy. Some humans seem to be more aware than others that it is seeking that underpins all human endeavor, and having become conscious seekers they make great efforts to create a life of experiences that hopefully reach their ideals of what is right.

A meaningful life for a seeker, whether or not a conscious seeker, is a life that lives up to the seeker's sense of what is the highest good, or most worthy of experiencing. And to make sure that we resist the simplistic view that physical pleasure is necessarily the highest good, I need to point out this sense of what is the highest good may not always be pleasurable. A martyr, for example, has the sense that dying for one's faith or cause is the most worthy available option and does so willingly, and arguably without enjoyment—at least in the sense of physical pleasure.

The desire for meaning in human life has long been recognized by people in different times and places, and systems and paths for the attainment of happiness or meaning have been drawn up to aid those who would benefit from the experience and wisdom of those who have gone before. Without their help, in fact, we would be forced to reinvent the wheel and travel down roads that others had discovered to be less than desirable, and perhaps even mortally dangerous. But with the help of maps of human experience and sense-making, we are empowered to pursue our activity with greater confidence, and attain greater experiences and discoveries of meaning.

So far so good. But a problem arises when we stop for a moment to consider our options. The human predicament, as human life has been called, is that life forces us, because of our self-awareness, to choose in each and every moment what the next step of our path will be. Even when we choose to do nothing, this is in effect a choice that will create further choices. There's just no getting off the bus.

What adds a further complication to this already complex situation is the fact that many of our choices are seemingly made for us. We are, if we choose to believe the investigations of our fellow humans and perhaps our own experiences, influenced by a collection of biological drives and psychological pre-dispositions and processes that function to varying degrees outside of our conscious awareness. And when we consider the big picture, it becomes dauntingly evident that we are inextricably linked and biased by all the choices ever made by ourselves, our parents, our cultures—and most of all by the grand sense-maker we sometimes call nature. We must admit that as self-aware as we may be, we are also enmeshed in the whole of life.

So once again it all comes down to the moment. In any given moment we are both bound and freed by all that has come before. And the choice is individually and repeatedly ours to make: will we consciously choose to step in a direction of greater transcendent meaning and happiness, or will we give ourselves over to be unconsciously swept up in the forces of sense-making that swell through us and around us in the grand dance we call life?

Either way, our lives will be rich in experience because experiencing life seems to be the root aim of consciousness. Even so, when we listen to the words and songs of humankind's greatest sages we will hear the advice that tells us to consciously open ourselves to the fullest meaning of our experience because it is intrinsic to life's design that in doing so we find our greatest happiness. In fact, there are repeated suggestions, and even emphatic insistence, that tell us that by consciously exploring ourselves and life we will discover that we are, in essence, Life itself.

Finding Our Way

But what if, as I suggested in the opening pages of this chapter, we have gotten something fundamentally wrong or are missing some vital information that keeps us from making the wisest choices for our happiness? For example, what if we don't realize that we must choose, with our hearts *and* our wills, to do our best to live the life that reflects our highest potentials for creativity and love? Or what if we don't understand that such a choice to live consciously means nurturing our emotional evolution and feeling things we've mistakenly learned to fear?

In other words, simply deciding to become fully and joyously alive isn't quite enough. We are individually and collectively masterpieces of complex display, and it is easy to become lost or stuck in the works. Even when we rely on the maps of our wise ones we discover that making sense of ourselves is not as straightforward as we might like. For one thing, much of what we are told about how to find greater meaning in our lives is confusing or paradoxical, and often there are blatant contradictions between maps or between what we are told and our own experience. When we add to this the likelihood that our own misperceptions and inner emotional wounding color our sense-making, we begin to grasp the enormity of the project we are taking on.

It is truly a life project we are talking about, and even considering it brings up an array of serious concerns. But whether we know it or not, we are in luck. By virtue of the very same complexity, design and diversity of life that often confounds us, we are already in possession of what we need to both guide and nurture us. In fact, there is nothing essential we will ever lack on this journey because it is the journey for which life has chosen and prepared us.

All that we will ever need will be available in the ever-present moment. This is because each moment is pregnant with our life's meaning, and as beings at the highly evolved end of nature's spectrum, we are dressed to the nines in the perseverance, courage, wit and compassionate understanding needed to perceive that meaning. It is indeed our greatest purpose to experience the transcendent truth of our lives, and so whenever we consciously take steps toward such greater authenticity, we are unfailingly met by the assistance we need. (It may not always be what we imagine we need, but it is always the most perfect guidance.)

Yet even with the certain assistance of life itself, we know from experience that some paths are more direct or more graceful than others. And experiencing the transcendent truth of our lives, we may also imagine, is something that seems to have been reserved for the most extraordinary humans—our sages and saints. We're more than willing to look to them for the direction we know we will need in order to minimize our wrong turns and to lighten the path before us, but most of us are not necessarily holding our breath for miracles.

But whatever our attitude concerning our chances for enlightenment or sainthood, accepting the gifts of experience from others, it seems clear, is a wise move. Yet without much investigation into the teachings of our extraordinary humans and the maps of our religions, wisdom traditions and philosophies, we come squarely across a significant contradiction; again and again we are told to stop looking outside of ourselves, that what we are looking for lives within us.

To a seeker there is probably no more frustrating message than the one which says that one should look no further, that all is already within one's grasp. It is nonetheless a profound truth, for if what is sought is divine meaning, joy or happiness, then this is necessarily a very personal matter. So what is needed, therefore, is a way for us to wisely interpret our experiences so that we may make greater sense of our lives and choose paths toward increasingly greater meaning and happiness.

Moreover, this wise approach to life will have to include a way for us to make sense of any and all experience, and it must also address the nature of experience so that we can learn to form a truly conscious partnership with life. And most of all, if it is to assist us in becoming fully human by guiding us to our transcendent truth, our understanding and approach to living must increase our experiences of joyous creation and love, which in our better moments we know (or at least suspect) in our heart of hearts to be the foundation of life.

A Practical Model for Perceiving Life

Perhaps the first thing we should know before we step blithely off into more of our personal adventures is just exactly where we, as humans, are in the overall scheme of things. And even before that, we need to understand that we are. These two things—where we stand and that we exist—are two fundamental aspects or faces of the same experience we call Life. (Capitalizing the word Life in this way serves to underscore not only that Life is greater than we are, but also that as conscious beings or creations of Life we share in its greatness.)

In fact the most basic way to understand what we call consciousness, which combines both where we are and the understanding that we exist, is to see consciousness as the degree to which a being interacts with and experiences Life. For example, and as mentioned earlier, humans have three modes of experience: body, emotion and mind, and these modes determine and reflect the degree of our interaction and experience of Life. And because our sole human activity and goal is to make sense of Life, a more complete understanding of consciousness is where we should begin. Of course we also need to keep in mind that the whole point of our quest is for the greater happiness that comes from emotional wisdom.

Human consciousness, as we know, differs from the other forms of consciousness with which we find ourselves keeping company. And when we apply the simple definition of consciousness as the degree of a being's interaction and experience of Life, we can readily see that we must grant consciousness status to all living beings— animals, humans and possibly even plants.

Such a definition of consciousness is somewhat different than what we might usually mean when we use the term, but this broad definition becomes necessary if we wish to recognize some important aspects and dynamics of the overall system or design of Life.

Also, this definition immediately points out that self-awareness or sentience in this model is not necessarily a pre-requisite for consciousness. Splitting hairs on the issue of what makes for sentience isn't required, though, because the overall point that there are clearly differences in consciousness among Earth beings is relatively self-evident, and it is this general, observable difference that is important for us to place ourselves in relation to our conscious cohabitants.

And regarding the placement of humankind in relation to other living beings, one relatively popular way of classifying Life on Earth is both general enough and accurate enough for our overall purposes. This is the traditional method of dividing Earth into four realms: mineral (or elemental), plant, animal and human. In terms of consciousness this seems rather reasonable because we can easily perceive a difference in the ways in which these groups or realms differ in their interactions with Life. At the same time, we should also apply our understanding of these four realms as interdependent and equally vital components in what's being called the web of life, or the living Earth. As we shall see, both of these concepts, distinct realms and holistic cooperation of the realms, are useful for the understanding of transcendence, which we shall soon need to discuss.

As important as it is to know that as humans we belong to the most highly evolved realm in terms of consciousness, it is even more fundamental for our purposes to understand what the differences in consciousness among the realms mean for us and our sense-making. The fact that we are even aware of ourselves to begin with is actually the first crucial piece of information that we can use to build upon to create a model or understanding of how we perceive Life. And understanding how we perceive Life will in turn go a long way in helping us not only to form a picture of Life, but also to understand then how to choose and evaluate our experiences. And if the model is sufficiently universal, if it can, in other words, be applied with success to all our perceptions, then we will be in a good position to perceive where we truly are—and in which directions we can find greater personal meaning and happiness.

To open this discussion, we should begin with the idea that self-awareness, or the knowledge that one exists, is a basic measure of a being's degree of consciousness. This is important to state because it provides a key to the purpose and function of consciousness, and therefore also to answering at least in a very basic way the question that has been known to confound seekers, and that is: Why Life? And from our perspective this question must be faced down right at the start, for without a satisfactory answer our journey will lack the inspiration and confidence we'll need to truly become fully human.

As it turns out, the question regarding the function and purpose of consciousness is not at all difficult to answer—nor is the answer to "Why Life?" especially troublesome. The real difficulty lies elsewhere—in how to implement and apply the implications of the answers. But that too can be dealt with once one has clarity of understanding, adequate tools, and purpose. So, back to the burning question: Why Life?

First of all, this is a question that must be answered in stages if we are to give it the kind of thoughtful consideration it demands. The first stage involves looking at what Life is showing and telling us by expressing itself as it does in degrees of consciousness—as is evidenced for example by the four realms. And from this evidence, and from the evidence now being provided by our life sciences (see Fritjof Capra's *The Web of Life* for an overview of this), we can see that Life works systematically to become aware of itself. The logic of consciousness, in other words, gives itself away as a holistic system intent on self-awareness. Without even having to place a value on self-awareness, we can witness that consciousness has a directional urge or drive, and this goal of consciousness is self-awareness.

Consciousness, in other words, can be understood to be a force. This can be seen simplistically in the workings of nature as the mineral beings nourish plant beings, and the plant beings provide food for more self-aware beings. Moreover, it is a self-sustaining system because the forms of the beings in the plant, animal and human realms are transformed back to the foundational or mineral realm after the force of consciousness has passed through them.

Or is the force of consciousness already present even in the elemental or mineral realm? If, as science and most religions and spiritual traditions point out, some kind of evolution is the system that defines or makes possible our urge for newness, diversity and growth, wouldn't we have to include the mineral realm as something more than an innocent bystander?

In the life sciences this means seeing life and the environment as co-creators or symbiotic partners. Our planet, in other words, can be seen as a single organism, with everything working together to maintain the life of the organism. This example gets right to the point that needs to be made from the start: when we speak of Life as intent on self-awareness through consciousness, we can not make any distinctions of forms that imply absolute separation because all forms are mutually interconnected and mutually interdependent. And so the statement that all realms are to some degree conscious seems to be just right around the next corner—which brings us in line with traditions such as some teachings of Native American spirituality that see all of Life as holy, and consequently bring forth the possibility for greater reverence in our lives.

Other traditions express this same idea of the mineral or elemental realm's intrinsic connection and cooperation with Life by identifying and categorizing these foundational elements. In the classical Western tradition, there are four elements whose qualities are seen to be underlying and constituting Life on Earth. They are identified as fire, water, earth and air. In other traditions there are different and sometimes more elements, such as the Chinese system, which identifies the five elements of water, fire, metal, wood and earth.

The important understanding to have is that these elements are not only representational of the mineral and plant realms, they are also symbolic; that is, they stand for the different qualities that the force of Life can assume—much in the same way the model categorizing four realms of being is a useful shorthand for considering the foundational faces of consciousness.

Before moving on to how self-aware consciousness actually works to produce a being's perception of its beingness, we should make a few more observations and additions regarding what has already been said. First of all, as another basic piece for the journey to discovering and living our greatest truth and therefore our happiness, the concept of consciousness also provides a convenient opening to a consideration of the process of transcendence, which is a natural characteristic or quality of Life. The seed becomes the tree, the water droplet becomes the snowflake, and the caterpillar becomes the butterfly—these are all poetic examples for the common but wondrous fact of Life's transcendent nature.

And from the model we're using that sees Life as a living system intent on self-awareness through consciousness, transcendence is the way in which the force of consciousness moves through the realms by changing or adapting form and increasing depth. To transcend means to go beyond, and in the case of the evolution of consciousness it also means that what has gone before is included in the next form (see Ken Wilber's works, such as *A Brief History of Everything*, for an in-depth discussion of this). This inclusiveness is an important distinction for the self-growth process inherent in our journey because it means that to really evolve we can't just move on, we have to move through and include, thereby increasing the depth of our experience. And since transcendence is the only way to greater self-awareness, which as we will see can only mean greater purpose, meaning and joy in our lives, we will have to learn how to recognize and work with transcendence in our everyday experience. To a large extent this will entail discovering the layers or depth of our being, especially the depths of our emotional nature.

At this point it is also interesting to mention at least briefly the difference between self-awareness in the human and animal realms (or any of the realms for that matter). Without getting bogged down by trying to postulate any exact measure, it should be enough for our purposes to conclude that it is the degree to which humans are capable of abstract reasoning and language that differentiates our self-awareness from the self-awareness of our animal realm companions. Dolphins, chimpanzees and other animals are self-aware, have language (and humor!), and are presumably capable of abstract thought, but not to the degree of humans. And this leads us quite neatly where we need to go next as we seek to become fully human and to answer the question of "Why Life?"

An Anatomy of Self-Awareness

As seekers, we should recognize the value in understanding just how our self-awareness arises, for the perception of self is the cornerstone of our sense-making. It is after all our self-awareness that gives us choice, and if our fundamental purpose and intention is to choose greater meaning and happiness for ourselves, then we need to know some details about how self-aware consciousness works. And we also require that this anatomy of self-awareness be in the context of Life as transcendent experience; otherwise we run the risk of not getting the whole picture. So to some degree we will have to leave the worlds of accepted psychology and brain science behind because they do not recognize how Life operates through a system intent on self-awareness, and that this intention is a big part of the answer to "Why Life?" Fortunately, at present there are many enlightened scientists and therapists implementing integral models of consciousness, and we will see much more of their work coming in to the mainstream of our culture in the coming years.

In the most basic terms, self-awareness is characterized by ego consciousness. What this means for humans is the use of "I" as point of reflective reference. Equally important is the consequence that awareness of self creates awareness of other, or non-self. Rational thought, it would seem, relies on the expression of one's self-awareness through some kind of language, and this sense of self immediately assumes or creates the concept of otherness.

This is related to what René Descartes considered the unassailable first position of true knowledge: "Cogito, ergo sum," or "I think; therefore I am." Descartes' statement points out that a consciously expressed awareness of the self is fundamental to a reasoning or imaginative being, for it creates an idea of self, an ego, that can be abstractly conceived and independently considered—as if it were *other*—and this in turn opens the way for all that is truly other or non-self to be separated, categorized, and abstractly manipulated.

Descartes' statement, however, is not a sufficient explanation of self-awareness (nor did he intend it to be) because it doesn't address the mechanics or anatomy of thought, and such an analysis is neces-

Dia. 1

sary for understanding how we make sense of things. As a step in that direction, we can use a simple diagram.

This diagram is a representation of the self-awareness associated with simple ego consciousness, which we can think of as the entry-level consciousness of humans. The circle should be understood to stand for the multi-dimensional sphere that encompasses all of the simple ego and non-self (other). It's also necessary to view the boundaries that separate simple ego self and non-self as fluid, changing according to the ego's conceptions of itself. This idea of a boundary or separation between simple ego self and non-self is important because it is the perception of separateness that characterizes the simple ego self.

Ego consciousness, in fact, requires the perception of separateness to create and sustain itself. In this light it is interesting to note that one of the first principles in many mystical and spiritual traditions is that separation is the primary illusion. And in our own experiences we have plenty of evidence to support this insight—especially when we consider the pathologies that result from the idea of separateness. One striking example is the degree to which humans destroy their own environment—as if humans could be separate from that environment.

Knowing that we exist may seem simple enough, but that apparent simplicity results from a masterful sleight of hand. Our sense of "I" requires us to take an imaginary step back from ourselves in order to conceive the sense of separateness. Of course it all happens so quickly and so out of our awareness that it's easy to miss. To slow down the process and analyze what goes on (in order to get a handle on how we perceive any experience), it is useful to think of human ego consciousness as a self-looping, holistic process involving the three modes of our experience (body, emotion and mind), and memory.

In order to grasp how this all works, we must first of all learn to accept that all of our experience is bound to and interconnected with our body or sensory experience. The term sensory experience, a vital step of the process of perceiving Life, is already something of a trick phrase because, as just mentioned, all experience is necessarily sensory. Our senses accept impressions of what it feels like to be alive, and these sensory impressions are included in all modes of our experience. Nothing, in fact, can be perceived by humans in an absolutely non-sensory way—try as we might to deny or forget our bodies and our emotions. All of our experience, even the most abstract mathematical thought, is grounded in sensory impression. To be human is to experience Life—in all its forms and aspects—through the senses because the modes of our experience are holistically interconnected (which is a fact we will later learn to use to our advantage for our journey to greater happiness).

There is of course a long tradition of denying the integral role of the body and the body's senses in all of our experience, and this tradition lives on in both Western and Eastern thought. It is imperative that we correct this misunderstanding, for the body and our physical senses offer us immediate access to deep layers of the psyche, thus affording us a means for transcending limiting beliefs, emotions and programming. Even when we consider the activity of Life that exists beyond the scope of our senses, for example when we speak for example of infrared light or radio waves, we conceive of such things in the terms of our senses. And if for the sake of argument we allow for the possibility or probability of receiving impressions or information from other dimensions, these impressions will necessarily also be perceived through (and colored by) the instruments of our senses. To deny this basic truth of our humanity, to attempt to bypass the body in any way, will ultimately prove to be self-limiting.

But the real key to our process for perceiving Life is memory. Memory, as the ability to store the information given by each of the modes of experience, is perhaps the true inspiration of self-aware consciousness, for memory is what allows us to hold an experience apart from itself. So maybe, with no disrespect to Descartes, it's more accurate to state: "I remember; therefore I am." Clearly the Greeks paid tribute to the importance of memory by having their goddess of memory, Mnemosyne, be the mother of the nine muses of inspiration in learning and the arts. Moreover, memory needn't be restricted to considerations of human consciousness. In a fashion, memory is an aspect of all of Life, from genetic coding to cell replication. But in respect to human self-awareness, the memory of experiences serves as the necessary precursor to how imagination or mind can make associations and create connections necessary for learning. And the fact that the forms or experiences of imagination can also be remembered is what births the genius of our minds.

In its importance to human self-aware consciousness, there is nothing greater than imagination, for it stands as the crown of our ability to know ourselves and choose greater happiness. This is because imagination or mind is the name given to the innate curiosity of our nature. Mind is the sorting, comparing and probing of memories and experiences to answer in some form the primary question of human self-awareness: Who am I? This question, in its larger conception, is nothing less than the question which lies at the heart of our sole activity of sense-making: What is Life? (These two questions are antecedents to the transcendent question already posed: Why Life?)

And to answer these basic questions of self-awareness, mind creates an image, a picture or an idea of whatever it turns its attention to—though we must be clear that our use of the word *image* does not restrict it to the visual sense. This image, in fact, is directly based on all sensory impressions and experiences of emotion and mind, and such images lead to understanding, including the understanding of self. The use therefore of imagination, as well of the interconnectedness of our modes of experience, allows us to be creative, heal and grow in surprising ways, as we will explore in later chapters.

Metaphoric Sense-Making

Simplifying the process of self-aware perception into the components of the three modes of experience and memory provides an insightful and manageable model for examining more closely how we make sense of things—especially how we make sense of our lives. At root of course in all of this is the fact that we are only able to make sense of things because there are satisfying and growth-inspiring answers to our basic question of "Who am I?" (or "What is Life?"), as well as to the transcendent question of "Why Life?" These questions and their answers reveal the order or design of Life, and the closer we come to understanding this order or design, the greater meaning and joy we experience and choose to experience.

One essential aspect of Life's design that becomes evident from a consideration of the process of human perception is that understanding comes from recognizing relationships. Thinking, feeling and reasoning, in other words, are associative. It is by associating one experience, thing or idea with another experience, thing or idea that we uncover or imagine the relationship that provides meaning. Understanding, in short, is metaphoric—we understand and know experiences, things and ideas only in terms of other experiences, things or ideas.

When you stop and consider this, you realize that it couldn't really be any other way. True separation, as mystics and quantum physicists tell us, is illusory. We live in a world of swirling, intermingling forms of energy to the degree that it's really not possible to say even where one thing ends and the next begins. Our sleight-of-hand perception of a separate self, or ego self, is likewise illusory; in a pure sense there is no real self and there is no real other. There is only Life. So within our all-encompassing world we make distinctions of self and otherness or *this* and *that* based on the differences and similarities we find in our perceptive senses of one thing or another. In other words, the process of self-aware consciousness lets us sort, organize and use our imaginations to probe—usually lightning fast and out of conscious awareness—for relative similarities and differences so that we can imagine and conceive our world of me and you.

The understanding that perception is metaphoric, or associative, is actually implied by its self-looping process of experience and memory. It is by grouping the sensations and characteristics of experiences (held in memory) that we make sense of them. Eating a piece of chocolate, for example, is an experience rich in sensory information from all five senses: sound, touch, taste, smell and sight. This information is collectively associated and helps form our experience of eating chocolate. The reason that it only helps and is not the full experience is because this chocolate-eating experience is further enhanced and given meaning by its relation to other experiences (including perhaps the craving for chocolate or memories of previous chocolate-eating experiences) that are being experienced or imagined in the same moment.

This, as you can see, could easily become a complicated and potentially confusing discussion if we wanted to map things out even further, but fortunately that's not necessary. For our purposes, a basic understanding of metaphoric sense-making is sufficient. Not only does it reveal the trick of consciousness that requires a sense of other in order to make associations, but it also shows us that our ways of thinking and understanding exist along a continuum of sorts, which means we have to rethink our ways of classifying ourselves and others into body, emotion or mind types. Human understanding and self-aware consciousness always involve all three modes of experience—though certainly it can be said that people develop themselves with preferences for one mode over the others.

What should also be made clear is that making these distinctions about our modes of experience, our process of self-awareness, and the metaphoric nature of our sense-making is important for one reason, and that is that it is useful to understand how we create our sense of self or identity so that we can focus on this book's main subject, which is emotional wisdom. Seeing where we are and how we operate, in other words, is only the foundation piece for our greater purpose, the journey to greater experiences and understandings of happiness and love.

The Matrix of Identity

In the same way that we associate experiences with other ones to form an understanding or conception, we create a complex arrangement, or matrix, of ideas (based on our experiences) in the creation of our mind's sense of identity. Matrix, as a word that comes from the Latin *mater*, or mother, actually means womb, and in mathematics a matrix is an arrangement of symbols. This is an interesting idea, that the arrangement of associative thoughts (which are in a very real sense symbols) we use to identify ourselves is a womb, a place where our birth is prepared. Such an idea is especially interesting in light of the understanding that we are more than our mind's ideas of ourselves, just as Life is vaster and grander than we could ever conceive. For what this implies, in essence, is that with every new idea or conscious experience of self we are born to an even greater self.

Such transcendence is the true way of self. This is because each matrix of self, as an ego or point of reference for self-aware consciousness, is a representation, a reflection, that continually moves, shifts and maps the path of our journey. But the water, as they say, is not the river. We are not our ideas of who we are any more than our reflection in the mirror feels the warmth of our bodies. In fact, it is when we believe that our ideas of ourselves are the whole picture that we run into trouble.

Ideas are largely static, so when we move through Life in the cloak of our mind's ideas of self we will eventually grind to a halt and get stuck. Ideas of self will eventually prove to be limiting because they will not, cannot, change and transcend themselves. For that we need emotion, because emotion is the gateway to our transcendence. Another way to phrase this is that mind cannot transcend itself; it can only make finer and finer distinctions based on associations. The heart, or emotion, on the other hand, is the vehicle for transcendence. So while the mind can take us to the point of inspiration in its associative imaginings, the actual leap of inspiration is a heartfelt, emotional experience. (This also makes sense in light of emotion's central position, energetically speaking, in the triad of our experiential modes.)

Perhaps the most striking consequence of this truth of the relationship between mind, transcendence and emotion is the way in which it rearranges what is meant by identity. For a variety of reasons that we will explore in later chapters, there is a tendency to believe that we are what we know of ourselves in our minds. What becoming fully human and choosing increasingly greater meaning requires, however, is that we identify with the transcendent self, for it is the transcendent self that is more fully integrated with emoti on—as well as with our inherent mystery—and therefore gifts us with awareness of our divine identity.

There is, in other words, usually quite a difference between our mind's conception of self and our authentic or divine identity, and this authentic identity is the one in full harmony with the design and purpose of Life—a design and purpose that is available for us to know and experience. Moreover, conscious identification with the transcendent self teaches us that the reality and wonder of our being is far more and goes much further than we usually ever imagine—to a large degree because we do not understand the role of emotion in our journey to greater self-awareness and personal meaning.

Before addressing how we come to know and experience the transcendent self and how it integrates our experience and allows us to grow into our potentials for love and creativity, it is important to reflect on how each of our modes of experience is incomplete and potentially faulty. In fact we are all familiar with the potentials for delusional imaginings, emotional overreactions and sensory illusions.

Especially the senses and sensory experience are given less than rave reviews when it comes to perceiving reality. Plato dealt with this in his "Allegory of the Cave," and it is also a long-standing teaching of Buddhism that the world of the senses is illusory. Indeed the view that the sensory world is not the real world is common to many teachings. But since our sensory experience is fundamental to how we make sense of the world, we need to make an important distinction: The senses, in and of themselves, are not illusory; it is how we interpret our sensory experience that determines its truth. The same could also be said for the other two modes of human experience. In fact, we need to establish our standard for truth if we claim that this or that experience or interpretation is potentially illusory. What, then, is our measure for truth?

Asking such a naïve or simplistic question is a sure way to be showered with knowing smiles from all the grown-ups in the room. Yet is there any more important question—especially in regard to identity? Don't we all wish to know the truth about who we are? And isn't such a quest for personal truth reliant upon having some standard or measure for truth?

Those who reply that there can be no absolute standard for truth, that truth is relative to a context or framework (such as the laws of physics or principles of mathematics—or even the dynamics of interpersonal relationships) seem to be on the right track somehow. Within such contexts we do find truths. But that kind of truth is nonetheless slippery; today's laws of physics will be overturned or at least deepened tomorrow, and even some of the so-called truths we discover about ourselves this week will become outdated before long.

So the problem with the context-dependent approach, though it works in the short-term, is that it does not encompass the overreaching context or framework within which everything happens. Nothing less than all of Life is our context, our framework for human meaning—and even though such a context can feel overwhelming, if we can find measures for truth in smaller contexts, it seems logical to assume that truth functions not only in relative, limited frameworks, but also in the whole experience we're calling Life.

We have to remember that this largest context possible, what we're calling Life, transcends our self-and-other consciousness, that sleight of hand that allows us to entertain the illusion of separateness. And from this vantage point, the universal measure for human truth is unconditional, universal love, for it is wholly life-affirming and celebratory in every moment. Again and again we have heard this message from our saints, sages and wise ones, and it is this perennial understanding of love's primacy that places emotion as the key mode of experience for our journeys into greater personal meaning and happiness.

Love, in other words, is the truth sense, the standard for determining what is most valuable in our lives. This concept or sense of truth will seem backwards to many, for we are so used to looking for our measures of truth from outside of ourselves, in what we sometimes like to call objective reality. Our sciences, in fact, see truth in this way, and within their contexts and frameworks they are completely right. Truth as a measure of personal meaning, however, will never be found outside of oneself because personal meaning is a matter of feeling, ultimately a feeling of happiness. And in the largest view perhaps, what we see and consider to be objective reality is the outer, observable expression of unimaginable joy and creative urge that is borne of the superlative self-aware consciousness that is the source of our being.

But however we choose to understand truth, we should be careful not to underestimate or even negate the importance of any of our modes of experience because of the belief that it is misleading or unreliable. Sense-making in all forms is logical, for the simple fact that logic is a reflection of the inherent metaphoric or associative design and order of Life. In human experience, therefore, there can really be nothing called pure logic if by pure logic we wish to say non-sensual. Similarly, emotion—often misunderstood as contrary to logic—is equally logical because emotion relies on the same sensory associations and imagination for its logic, and these relationships of meaning mirror an order or matrix that both precedes and has fashioned human consciousness.

Recognizing that all modes of human experience are on the same logical continuum of sense-making has great bearing on the identification of the transcendent self. Body, emotion and mind work together, in fact, to create and fine tune the matrix of identity. Mind works from a relative critical distance, coolly making sense of the big picture. This is reflected by our linguistic choice to have "to see" mean to understand—sight is the sense that extends farthest from the here and now feelings of the body.

Emotion, on the other hand, works from within these feelings and how they directly express and affect our sense of being. Correspondingly, emotion is linked with the sense of touch, and we speak of being emotionally moved, or "touched." As representations of Life, all modes of human experience are alike in their richness and complexity, but their differences are what allow us to identify and make sense of our personal stories. And story, as the blended emotional, psychological, intellectual and physical sense-making of our personal experience, is the realm of the transcendent self.

A Quest for Meaning

Life unceasingly questions, explores and creates, so we are only following our deepest impulses when take up the questioning, exploring and creating that is Life's business. We constantly ask ourselves and others questions in order to help us decide what to do next in our never-ending quest to find and sustain happiness in our lives. We could even say that because our sole activity is to make sense of Life, that Life poses itself to us as a question, or even three basic questions: "Who are You?"; "What is Life?"; and "Why Life?" (or "What's Life's purpose and value?").

As it turns out, of course, not all of the answers we have to these questions are conscious, and not all of them are in harmony and agreement with Life's purpose and design for us, which is for us to find and reach our greatest potentials for love and creativity. And while it may not be possible to have a wholly wrong answer to any one of these three basic questions posed by Life, some answers are certainly better than others for gracefully finding the path of greater personal meaning and happiness.

Given that not all of the answers we have to these questions are conscious, and some of our conceptions of Life are faulty or incomplete, how do we know when we've hit upon the right answers? The short answer to this question is relatively simple: We know we have correctly answered any specific question posed by Life when we become greater—when we transcend our own conception of our self and become more unconditionally loving.

This is in fact what it means to identify with the transcendent self. Life is and will always be greater than an individual perception of it, and the transcendent self accepts and seeks greater identification with the design and purpose of Life. That is why it is so important that we know how to make sense of our experience (through all three modes) in ways that clarify how Life is guiding and shaping us to our highest.

At this juncture we also need to finally do more than imply an answer to the question "Why Life?" Having love as the measure of truth provides the key, for love is therefore also the highest experience and purpose of Life—as well as the answer to our question. And before you close the book or your mind in response to this explosion of naïveté, let me make clear that having love as the value, purpose and truth of living does not mean that our lives are meaningless if we're not blissed out on love all the time.

Quite the contrary. The scale of possible love in Life is virtually unimaginable, just as we cannot grasp the number of worlds that populate our heavens. That our lives are full of trials and suffering doesn't change the fact that the measure of truth is love, though it may shift our understanding of suffering. The relative understanding of the scope and possibility of our experience may also begin to open our eyes to the scale of Life, and the wonder of our own being. And as seekers of our identity and truth this is important, for we need to know the overall lay of the land.

Our quest for meaning, in essence, is ultimately a quest for the love of life and living creatively that lies at the heart of the experience of the transcendent self. Furthermore, consciously engaging our quest by testing our answers to Life's questioning will provide a personal map for identifying in which directions lie greater experiences of meaning and transcendence—and therefore love. This process of inquiry, in effect, is the navigational link between what we already know and experience of Life and our personal growth or transcendence. One insightful way to think of this is to see any question that we have about our personal meaning as a reflection or mirror image of Life's basic inquiry: "Who are You?" This is a very useful understanding, for it helps us know how to create a personal process of inquiry that reflects and is therefore in harmony with Life's design.

Dia. 2

Of course the basis for such an exploration of how and where we can locate the areas for transcendence in our lives should be the understanding of how we perceive ourselves and create our sense of identity. In these diagrams the difference between the simple ego self or conditional consciousness and the transcendent self or unconditional consciousness is illustrated.

It is immediately apparent that this second diagram is reminiscent of the human eye and its dark center, the pupil. This is a useful analogy, for it highlights a basic difference between the simple ego self, which sees other, or non-self, as external, and the transcendent self, or true self, which recognizes that other is both outer and inner. Indeed the primary difference between the simple ego self and the transcendent self is that the transcendent self recognizes that the impulse or force of its being is linked with the eternally unknown (mystery)—represented in the diagram by the dark sphere in the center. This reflects that the true nature of self is the nature of becoming, or in other words that its essence is always involved with its potential (or that which has not yet become).

In all of this it is important to keep in mind what may at first appear to be a paradox: Becoming is always in the moment. "Who am I?", "What is Life?" and even "Where do I go from here?" are all questions that lead to the experience of the moment. In one sense, finding personal meaning in the moment is a matter of recognizing the present form of Life's questioning and choosing or creating an answer. We therefore need to know how to recognize the questioning, as well as how to ask appropriate questions that will result in an answer or choice of greater meaning. The explorations of emotional development and healing that follow will hopefully do just that.

We also need to keep in mind that the essential nature of transcendence implies that whatever answers we give or choices we make will always become part of a new form of Life's questioning. What remains eternal and unchanging, however, is the energetic source of Life: a love of living that overflows in its creation of new forms for expressing and displaying such love. So as we turn our attention now to making sense of our emotional journey, we should do so with the intention of finding ways to more consciously and effectively create our lives to be in harmony with Life's love of living that is our purpose and highest potential for happiness.

Chapter One Main Points

1.   The three modes of human experience—body, mind and emotion—are holistically interwoven. Application: Favoring one or more of these modes at the expense of the other(s) indicates an imbalance that limits one's ability to create an authentic life.

2.   *Now* is the only true experience we ever have, and therefore the most real we can get. Application: We can not change the past; we can only change our present relationship to it to reveal what energies are present and available for transformation.

3.   Making sense of our personal lives, and of life in general, is the sole activity of human existence. Application: When we recognize how much our beliefs are formed by unconscious acceptance of our culture's responses to the universal question of what life is all about, then we take steps toward personal empowerment.

4.   Life works systematically to become aware of itself. Application: Knowing that the force of consciousness that works through us also works to support us in our quest to become more divinely awake creates trust for the evolutionary process of our spirit.

5.   Transcendence is the way of the force of consciousness, which means that what has gone before is included in the new form. Application: Our transcendent way of growth requires us to embrace the mystery of our becoming.

6.   Ego consciousness, or having an I-perspective, requires the perception of separateness to create and sustain itself. Application: Understanding that simple egoC consciousness is based on the idea of separation gives us insight into our feelings of separation and loneliness.

7.   All of our experience is grounded in sensory impression. Application: Recognizing that mind, body and emotion are truly inseparable opens the way for us to find balance.

8.   Understanding is metaphoric; we understand and know experiences, things, and ideas only in terms of other experiences, things
or ideas. Application: Personal growth relies on making sense of our
present experience within a context of positive change.

9.   Emotion is the gateway to our transcendence. Application:
Our ideas of ourselves, others and Life can limit our emotional evolution if those ideas are inflexible.

10.   The universal measure for truth is unconditional love. Application: This means that emotion is the key mode for our journeys
to greater personal meaning and happiness.

Exercise for Experiential Understanding

This exercise demonstrates the interactions and interconnections
of your three modes of experience (body, emotion and mind). You
will need paper, a pen or pencil, and colored pencils or crayons.

Once you have found a comfortable place to be undisturbed for
at least 20 minutes, take a few moments to breathe deeply and relax.
Pay special attention to your body, feeling in to where whatever you
are sitting or lying on presses up against you. Next, recall an unpleasant experience you remember from your past. Visualize it as
best you can, remembering sensory details. Once you have brought
the memory into your present awareness for at least one full minute,
pay attention for a minute or so only to the emotional feelings that
have been evoked. Don't analyze, just feel and observe. Next, pay
attention to what you are feeling in your body, and make a note of
any sensations or discomforts. When you have finished scanning
your body, with the colored pencils or crayons make an abstract drawing of the feelings that were evoked. Take your time, allowing yourself
to simply draw intuitively, from the inside out.

Once you have made your drawing, see if you can make sense of how your physical sensations, the story, and your emotions all fit together. What do you think are the connections between your remembered unpleasant situation and the physical sensations you noticed? Why did you choose the colors you did? Does your drawing's shape or shapes remind you of anything? Do your current reactions to the memory of your chosen unpleasant experience surprise you? Do they suggest connections to other memories?

To close: take a few moment to reflect on how this experience has changed, even slightly, your sense of that unpleasant experience in relation to your current idea of who you are. How have you changed? Is this a change that has just happened, or are you simply now more aware of a change that had already taken place? How does this change shift your personal sense of identity, if at all?

Questions for Contemplation

To what degree am I consciously doing my best in each of the three spheres of my life: health, relationships, and work? Where do I settle for surviving rather than creating conditions where I can flourish? (Note: lack of motivation or inspiration is an issue of *depth*. When we are not inspired by our lives, this is an indication of emotional issues that we are either unaware of or consciously avoiding.) Try using the Exercise for Experiential Understanding above (or use Chapter 4's) to peel back layers and bring forth emotional issues holding you back from living your real life.

Notes:

The Human Emotional Journey

The idea of emotion as a reliable path to the truth turns out to be far less objectionable, and becomes perhaps even rather obvious, when we accept unconditional or universal love as the measure or standard for personal truth. Love, as the highest form of our happiness, is our greatest good. We all wish to be happy, and wish for those we love to be happy, and on our best days we want everyone in the world to be as happy as humanly possible.

In fact, as diverse and unique as we all are, in our heart of hearts we are all yearning for the same things: above all, to be approved of and loved for who we are; and then to use our creative talents to serve others and for our own pleasure. This, of course, is the way of universal love. Such love only wants for all to experience and enjoy love. We can therefore say that in a very real sense our deepest desire is a kind of universal truth. In essence, we each want what everyone wants. With love, in other words, the personal is revealed to be universal.

But even if we stay within the bounds of the personal, and consider our deep desire for love on its own merits, we see that our highest good or truth is a highly emotional experience. This means that the key mode of our human experience is emotion. Our other modes of experience, the physical and mind, are equally essential to our overall human journey, but emotion and emotional experience must be recognized as the inspiring force of our evolution toward increasingly greater experiences and understandings of love and creativity (which can be understood as the activity generated by love). This perspective not only clarifies the paths we are on, individually and collectively, but it also opens up a way for us to better understand our interactions with Life, as well as the dynamics of Life's design or system for guiding and shaping us to our highest potentials.

This idea that heart wins out over mind when it comes to making our wisest choices can still be a tough sell, however. We are so used to relying on our minds to figure out the best possible choice or to calculate the odds for success that we can easily lose sight of the fact that our highest goal, which is our happiness (and of course the happiness of those we love), is an emotional experience. And for the most part, our hesitation about putting emotion first can be readily justified. We all have plenty of examples to draw from where doing exactly just that landed us in troubled waters, and once burned, we're twice shy.

Which is exactly right. When we get hurt, that's usually a clear sign that something's wrong, and the greater the hurt, the greater the wrong. In one sense, pain is both the definition and experience of *wrong*. What we often don't get right, however, is why a choice we thought we had made for our greatest happiness turned out to be the cause for pain. Getting an overview of the journey and dynamics of human emotional development will go a long way toward empowering us to make the kinds of choices that will in fact increase our experiences of positive emotions. This is because our journey toward universal love makes sense of all emotion, pleasant and unpleasant.

Practicing the art of emotional wisdom requires some fundamental understandings—we must be familiar with the basic outline of the journey of human emotional development, we must recognize the emotional forces and dynamics that make up our being, and we must also understand how to best work the ways in which mind, body and emotion commingle and interact.

In this chapter we will first of all make sense of the human emotional journey, including its evolutionary dynamics, and then we will examine more closely how mind, body and emotion work together. In that discussion we will also introduce how our beliefs and stories can both mask and reveal our emotional wounds, which is a topic that will be explored in greater detail in later chapters. Chapter Three will then take a look at the film *The Wizard of Oz* as a living cultural myth for the transcendent journey. This will allow us to put everything we have covered all together (and to have some fun!) before focusing more intently on what is specifically involved in emotional healing, personal growth, and your life's creative work.

Evolutionary Emotional Dynamics

Just as a newborn child is one hundred percent physically dependent upon its parents, that same child is also completely emotionally dependent. In fact a child's core needs for safety, nurturance and guidance reflect this dependency for all modes of the child's experience, whether physical, emotional or imaginative. (Note how each of these core needs has a mode correlate: body for safety, nurturance for emotion, and guidance for mind.) And a child whose core needs are not met, or are insufficiently met, will have a difficult if not seemingly impossible time reaching emotional maturity, which is a level of development essential for true, lasting happiness.

It is this journey from emotional dependency to emotional maturity that we must therefore be most concerned with in our search to realize our potentials for love and creative expression. Each of us travels our own version of this path, with varying success, but even if our emotional journey starts off on less than ideal ground, as is almost certain, we can still manage to live the life of our greatest potential. In fact, as we shall see, the emotional wounding that inevitably occurs in childhood and adolescence can act not only as the way-shower, but also as the energetic source for our eventual emotional flowering. Another way to say this is that our emotional wounding reflects our potential, and is in some sense the drive we feel to evolve emotionally.

The place to start, though, is with whether or not we believe Life to be benign. In the most basic sense, any understanding of our initial emotional dependence and how it functions in our overall human emotional development will be determined or at least highly affected by whether or not we believe Life to be fundamentally good. This is in fact the keystone, the leverage point, for virtually all personal growth, and it is best to get it out in the open before going any further.

After all, it only makes sense that our underlying core belief about the nature of Life's intention for us or relationship to us will shape how we see ourselves and our world—and consequently determine what choices we see available to us. Later we will look much more specifically at the different forms of this core belief, but for now we should at least be aware that this belief forms a distinct crossroads for wherever we are to go next in our life's journey.

Actually, the notion that Life is benign is an implicit assumption of the understanding we've already reached: that happiness is what our search is all about. We seek happiness through the experiential process of our self-awareness, as discussed in the last chapter, and this, at the very least, means that greater and greater happiness is our highest potential.

From there it is no great leap to consider that since the direction of the force of consciousness is toward self-awareness, and since the experiential process of our self-awareness is centered around or designed to draw us toward increasingly greater happiness, that the basic design or intention of Life, as the context for consciousness and self-awareness, is about our finding and realizing such happiness. This makes Life undeniably benign—even when we don't necessarily get all the whys and hows.

So with Life's basic goodness established as the foundation for how we can understand our emotional journey or evolution from emotional dependency to emotional maturity (and perhaps from there to emotional enlightenment), we need to turn our attention to the dynamics of this process. And this begins with the fact of our initial emotional dependence.

We are all born into a world that must meet our basic needs for physical and emotional sustenance if we are to have any chance for survival, and this relationship to our surroundings sets up the dynamics for the first leg of our journey. As for possible reasons for this, within the overall context of Life's benign intention or relationship with us, at this point we have to simply be satisfied with the position that our evolution to greater happiness begins with emotional dependence because in some way that arrangement serves the needs of that evolution. This is of course begging the question to some degree, so later we will explore some specifics of how this makes sense in a larger context.

Actually, our emotional relationship to our world begins in the womb, as we absorb the emotional energies of our mothers along with the food and everything else that we share. And of course that's only the beginning. After birth we are reliant upon and absorb the emotional energies of our fathers, as well as other caretakers, siblings and any extended family, as we learn to have emotional relationships. These emotional relationships in fact reach beyond people to any and all relationships we have with our surroundings, as is clearly evident in the magical thinking stage of children where the faces and changes of nature are emotionally related to. Dark skies are angry, flowers are happy, and raindrops are tears.

Emotional bonding for an infant is clearly foundational in her or his overall development. This is important to understand because it points to the primacy of our emotional mode of experience over the mind mode of experience in our relations with others and our world. In fact it may even be possible to state that just as the body mode of experience is primary to the development of emotional relationships, the emotional mode of experience is primary to the development of the mind. In any case, as we shall see, the relationship between mind, body and emotion is thoroughly interdependent.

Idealization

One vitally important dynamic in our emotional growth and evolution that occurs during the emotional dependency stage of our journey is the idealization process. Each of us idealizes our parents or primary caregivers. Perhaps this comes from the fact of our physical dependence. In other words, since we are physically dependent upon our parents to provide for us, which they do or we simply don't survive, we emotionally bond with them. This bonding then leads us to idealize them. They are good, or the greatest, because they provide us with our core needs for safety, nurturance and guidance. Or perhaps it is even more basic than that. We idealize them because having our needs met, even mostly, feels good, and we then associate feeling good with the ones who seemingly provide us with this goodness. We are made to feel good, and this means *they* are good.

Of course we are referring here to the best case scenario; in reality there are plenty of things that can go wrong in terms of having these core needs met. Interestingly enough, however, idealization can be heightened by less than ideal conditions. A child who knows hunger can come to appreciate the parents who alleviate it—even sporadically, thereby strengthening idealization. If abuse of any kind is involved, there can quickly develop confusingly strong contrary emotions that must coexist somehow in the child's sense making of the world it inhabits.

In any case, to some degree or another we all idealize our parents, and this idealization process is important for how we will grow and emotionally evolve. In the overall context of Life's design, the idealization process serves two needs at once, which in a larger sense are actually the same need. When we idealize our parents, the intensity of that emotional relationship anchors in all the emotional energies we have absorbed from them, and these emotional energies (or emotional relation patterns if you prefer) then literally become a part of who we are.

Of course we have our own temperaments and our own experiences, but into that mix is added whatever we have experienced of our parents' emotional energies. And those energies or relational patterns connect us to our grandparents and great-grandparents, and so on down the line. From the perspective of the overall emotional evolution of humankind, this passing on of emotional energy is as vital as the passing on of DNA, for it makes sure that we collectively work out the emotional tensions as well as take in the gifts of emotional wisdom of our families.

The other half of this equation is that such emotional inheritance also sets the stage for our individual evolution as well. The simple reason for this is that we are not our parents, and our human journey is largely about finding and expressing our unique identity. And the degree to which we can successfully claim or create our authentic selves is directly related to how well we manage to work through the tensions of our emotional inheritance in a way that supports and encourages that creation of our own unique being. Of course there are many other factors involved in our emotional development—including the emotional realities of the cultural institutions that shape us—but there is probably no greater influence than the emotional inheritance that is anchored in by the emotional idealization of our parents or primary caregivers.

The Essential Evolutionary Dynamic

In addition to our initial emotional dependence and the emotional idealization of our parents, there is a deeper facet of our emotional development that not only connects us to the transpersonal or universal aspects of our identity but also drives us to evolve. This is the deep inner knowing or sense of our absolute interconnectedness to all of Life, which in emotional terms can be understood as our intrinsic sense of undeniable worthiness. We are all children of God, or offspring of Life, and this validates our right to exist equally alongside all other creations.

Such deep inner knowing of our complete interconnectedness can be taken one step further: as self-aware beings we can become aware that we are participants in God's or Life's creating, and this participation implies that in some sense we are in fact God or Life. And the deep inner awareness of this truth of our divinity, whether we speak of it as soul awareness or whatever, is the foundation of the essential dynamic that inspires us to make choices that will bring us closer and closer to consciously living and experiencing that truth.

A dynamic, of course, suggests motion or movement, and in our emotional make-up this motion is created through tension. In simple terms, dynamic tension for our emotional evolution is provided by the interplay between the deep inner knowing that we are unconditionally divine, and the conditionality that we experience in our humanity. More specifically to the point, the deep foundational truth of our unconditional divinity is repeatedly confronted by our conditional experiences of identity. And it is identity, as we shall see, that serves as the true vehicle for our emotional evolution as we struggle to make sense of what this dynamic puts into play.

We can easily get a sense for what this means for the creation of our ego, our reference point of identity, by looking at how approval is a key component of our development. As much as our parents and caregivers may strive to unconditionally love us all at times, there are also conditional tests of approval that we undergo from an early age: to get approval, we must act or be a certain way. Naturally, a large part of this is to assist us so that we may develop the life skills and independence we will need to survive and thrive in the world, but there will of course also be elements of our parents' own emotional wounding that will go into whether or not we receive approval. And it doesn't begin and end with our families either; we are constantly being confronted by our cultures and institutions to behave or be certain ways in order to find approval.

Of course this dynamic is an essential part of Life's design. Our emotional journey begins in dependence and winds toward emotional maturity, which is not independence but a mutual interdependence that requires that we have learned to be responsible to make choices that will ensure that our basic needs for safety, nurturance and guidance are met. And since it is only from the place of true emotional maturity that we will reach our potentials and find satisfying and empowering relations with others and the world, it is wise for us to understand how and why this core emotional dynamic works in our choice and sense-making.

That the inner life is where we should turn in our quest for peace, love and enlightenment is something that we are told again and again by our religions and by our greatest sages. The Buddha instructed his followers to turn inward in the search for uncovering one's true self, as did Jesus when he said that "the kingdom of God is within." In fact every age and every wisdom tradition finds some way to repeat this perennial truth—even Hollywood, as we shall see when we take a close look at *The Wizard of Oz* in the next chapter. And in emotional terms, what we find when we turn within is an identity struggle, fueled by the tension generated by the reality of our unconditional worthiness as it meets the inauthentic condition-ality imposed by the false and incomplete belief systems of our egos.

The fact of this universal human identity struggle immediately raises two questions. The first one is, "What, in the overall context of Life's design, is the purpose or function of our identity struggle?" The second question is, "What can we do to resolve or reduce the tension of this struggle?"

Naturally, finding answers to the first question will go a long way toward answering the second one. And neither question can be an-swered without accepting and seeking to understand another of the perennial truths offered to us by our religions and wisdom traditions, and that is that our human lives are framed and fashioned by suffer-ing. Turning once more to Buddhism and Christianity, we find that suffering, and redemption from suffering, are central to the teach-ings. In Buddhism it is taught that desire is the source of our suffering, and that learning to free ourselves from attachment to our desires, as did the Buddha, will set us on the course to peace and happiness. In Christianity the lesson is similar: suffering is both inherited (as in original sin) and comes from going against the laws of God (or Life); and redemption is found through placing God's will for us above our own fears and desires—as exemplified in the crucifixion and resur-rection of Jesus.

Buddhism and Christianity, in other words, share the view that suffering comes from the misguided belief that we know what we truly want and what is best for us. We think our desires are what we want, but according to Buddhism, these desires are what cause suf-fering. We think we know what is best for us, but according to Christianity, we are best off when we surrender to God's will. And in both cases we can see the essential identity dynamic at work, which is the struggle between our unconditional self and the conditioned or conditional self of the ego. In truth, we are not our desires, as

Buddhism rightly teaches, and just as Christianity teaches, we must surrender our false sense of self so that our authentic identity can be revealed to us.

One reason for our relative ignorance about this inner struggle for authenticity is that we don't understand human emotional evolution, and we don't understand how body, emotion and mind function together, in concert with Life, to promote our evolution. This means first of all that we must learn to see the purpose in our identity struggle from the largest possible context, and from that begin then to grasp how we can ease or resolve the suffering of our struggle.

Toward Emotional Maturity

Just as we have said that consciousness is a force intent on self-awareness, we can say that this same force works through us emotionally to take us from emotional dependence to emotional maturity. We must, in other words, wean ourselves from emotional dependence on our families and culture (including our institutions) so that we can not only be self-aware, but also so that we are emotionally free to enter into relationships of unconditional integrity with others and with our world. The reason for this is that it is only through mutually supportive and mutually honoring relationship that our potentials for love and creativity can be realized. This declares of course that beyond emotional dependence is not separation or disconnection, but richer emotional experiences and greater connection.

Emotional maturity primarily means becoming responsible for making the choices that will ensure that our basic needs for safety, nurturance and guidance are met, and met in mutually unconditional ways (win/win). This will create the conditions for what

Abraham Maslow called self-actualization, which is the flowering of our uniqueness and creativity in such a way that it supports us while serving others. In later chapters we will go through this more thoroughly. For the moment, we must first of all understand that this journey to emotional maturity is ideal for our reaching our potential as loving, creating beings, and also recognize that our fuller understanding of the emotional evolution process will clarify our struggles with our authentic identity so that we can consciously assist the process of our emotional evolution. This will ease and eventually resolve much if not all of the suffering in our lives.

To that end, we now have to explore in a basic way what happens next, following the emotional idealization of our parents and caregivers. As you'll recall, this idealization process makes certain that we completely internalize the emotional energies or patterns of our parents, which has the purpose of ensuring not only our emotional evolution as a species but also our individual emotional evolution. This is because as individuals we seek at all times our greatest happiness, which at this early stage of our emotional development means being accepted and approved of by our parents. Quite quickly of course this desire to be accepted and approved of extends out into the world of family, teachers, authority figures and eventually work, but always the foundational level of our emotional identity will be shaped in large part by the relationships we had with our parents during early childhood.

The basic identity struggle between our unconditional worthiness and our conditional humanity is also going on from this very early age, even if only on a subconscious level. It's almost as if we begin to unconsciously notice that our parents and other people don't always recognize us as the best thing that's ever happened. And from that point on the formation of our conditional identity or ego is assured.

In order to ease the tension between the truth of our unconditional worthiness and the conditional approval that is being reflected back to us by the world, we start to shape ourselves and our identities in order to maximize approval of any sort. This means that we act one way with one person to gain maximum approval, then another way with another or others, and later for approval from our peers and society we may perform all kinds of contortions. (Naturally we do this to varying degrees, depending on temperament and personal history.)

One result of all this self-shaping we do is compartmentalization. We segment ourselves and our identities into personality packages that are designed to gain us maximum acceptance and approval. Such compartmentalization, however, leads to decreased energy, as well as relationships where we broker (usually unconsciously) one kind of approval for another instead of holding to the truth of our authentic identities. And conflicts, of course, are inevitable whenever we enter into conditional relationships, even (or especially) when such relationships are with ourselves. This is due to the power of the truth of our absolute worthiness. In fact, emotional wounding is exactly that: the painful tension that results from the formation of any conditional identity over the unconditional identity of our absolute divinity.

So why do we accept such lies about who we are in the first place? The obvious answer is that the force of our conditioning is simply overwhelming, and most of the significant conditioning occurs before we can even try and reason things out for ourselves. And then throughout our lives, wherever we turn we are faced with messages and reflections of our conditional worthiness. Receiving love and approval means doing and being what others or society expect from us; and this is quite often for us to meet *their* needs, not really for our needs, or for our highest mutual needs, to be met. In a basic sense, love or approval is generally perceived to be a limited commodity, and there's a mad scramble to get whatever brand of it you can—almost at any cost.

Yet since we are all unconditionally worthy, there's a deeper reason for why we accept the lies of our conditional worthiness than simply "that's the way the world works." After all, humans created our society, and they did so based on the realities and dynamics of human emotional development. In fact later, in our explorations of work and creativity, we will have to draw several important conclusions about where we are as a society based on the kinds of relations that we currently have with each other and our world.

For now, however, it is important to see that what underpins our relations with others and the ways in which we learn to give power to the conditional identity we are calling ego or simple ego (as opposed to the concept of the transcendent ego introduced earlier) is how the idealization of our parents and caretakers contributes to an emotional identification with conditional ideas and beliefs of our identity and worth.

The way this works is quite simple, though the results can be quite varied and complex. Having emotionally idealized our parents for their meeting of our needs and for the love they show us, as we begin as adolescents to establish some measure of autonomy from them, and therefore a sense of independent self, we quickly come face to face with the reality that they will not be able to meet all of our needs. This is of course as it should be, so that we can grow into emotionally mature beings, but it is nonetheless a difficult truth that directly touches the core of the emotional wounding created by our identity struggle.

In truth there is but one emotional wound, and all of the varieties and forms of emotional wounding are different faces of this one wound at the core of our emotional being. Whenever we feel we are not recognized (or whenever we do not recognize ourselves) for the truth of our absolutely unconditional worthiness, we will experience emotional pain. And this pain drives our choices because it is the purpose of our journey to be seen and to see ourselves for who we truly are—because that is where we will find our greatest happiness. So when it dawns on us, consciously and unconsciously, that first of all our parents and then the world around us can not or perhaps refuses to see the truth of our being, we experience the pain of this core emotional wound.

The outer form and expression of this wounding is anger, and it is often present even when not expressed (though the body will always show unexpressed anger in some form—such as fatigue or disease). We are angry that we are not being seen and treated for who we are. We feel unwanted, misunderstood, neglected—and all the other emotions of separation from truth. This kind of anger is seen especially during adolescence, when the pressures for finding and declaring one's sense of self are quite high. But as we know, anger is not restricted to adolescence. The pain of our separation from the truth of our being can be felt during any stage of life, and the greater the anger, the greater the concentration of the pain we are feeling. And of course anger can take many forms, including frustration, annoyance, bitterness, cynicism and rage, anger's most concentrated form. In fact any time we feel that we are being treated unjustly—either by others or by Life—we will feel some form of anger.

But anger is only the shell, the outer-directed energy of our core wounding. The deeper essence and reality of this wounding is self-diminishment, which is the inner-directed energy that keeps the wounding alive. And like anger, self-diminishment has many forms, ranging from self-negation to self-loathing. Also, it should be understood that anger and self-diminishment are an energetic pairing; you can't have anger in any form without there also being a form of self-diminishment present. This is because in reality self-diminishment is the source of anger in all its forms.

The Inner Lie

Perhaps what Christianity calls original sin and what Buddhism and Hinduism calls karma is tied in, at least in part, to the emotional idealization process. For once we have internalized the emotional energies of our parents and caretakers, and then idealized them for how they meet our basic needs and love us, we have unwittingly played into the basic human drama of lack.

The beginnings, or opening scenes, of this drama are inspired by the completeness of our idealization. Having created perfect gods and goddesses of our parents (or confused god/demon pairs in abuse cases), we are immediately in a bit of a bind when things do not go our way. We are of course unconsciously in touch with the deep inner knowing of our divinity, but faced with the physical and emotional power imbalances of childhood, we will naturally take these realities to be more convincing. And when we add to our emotional idealization the fact that we have internalized the emotional energies of our parents (which will include the patterns of their core wounding), what happens is that we feel that something about us must be lacking—otherwise we would be catered to for the satisfaction of all our needs and wants!

These emotional dynamics are unavoidable. Our human journey for the realization of our potentials for love and creativity means going from emotional dependence to emotional maturity, and perhaps even to emotional enlightenment. This requires that we learn from the inside out who we are and what we need, and Life's strategy for that involves the evolutionary dynamic that forces us to learn that in every moment we have a choice between the lie of our conditional worthiness and the truth of our divine, unconditional worthiness. In order to find peace and happiness we must learn, in other words, that in truth we lack nothing, for we are always all of who we need to be.

That the basic human drama revolves around lack can be seen by how we allow and empower our conditional identity, what we are calling the ego, to try and control Life. Feeling and fearing that we will never get enough, or never be enough, or never be seen for how truly wonderful we are, we scramble around in our insecurity, hoping to arrange things *just so*. Our misguided belief is that once we have things arranged just the way we want them, the suffering that characterizes our lives will stop, or at least be greatly reduced.

If we could only have *x* amount of money, or have *this* kind of job or marriage, then everything would be perfect—or so we believe. This kind of controlling attitude, however, will only lead to more disappointment and suffering because the desire to control Life stems from our deepest wound—the one that tells us that we are not already good enough in every way. Such an attitude also blinds us to the realities of how Life is working to shape and guide us to our most creative form. Convinced of our unworthiness, we fail to recognize how we are being shaped to bring forth the beauty of our potential being—and this is what prevents the realization of our greatest gifts.

Moreover, it's fairly clear to see how the drama of lack characterizes how we run our society—especially since all choices we make are in some way emotional decisions affected by our degree of core wounding. The sun, wind and water of our world provide all the inexhaustible energy we could ever need, yet we choose in our fearful lack-mindset to continue to have a conditional and exploitative relationship with our world's resources that causes us to create energy systems that deplete us and endanger the safety of our world. We are all beings of extraordinary beauty and grace, yet we agree upon narrow definitions of physical beauty that create a widespread sense of lack, of never being able to measure up. In these and other ways, our human society reflects back to us how inadequately we understand and know how to work with the inherent tensions of our becoming self-aware, unconditionally loving and creative beings. Our human society also reflects back to us just how deeply our core wounding is buried in our ideas about the meaning and purpose of our lives.

In short, it would appear that authentic emotional maturity is an ideal that is rarely modeled to us in our families and in our societies. Unclear and uncertain about who we really are, we become hypnotized by the controlling ways and beliefs of ego, which are fear- and lack-based, and this prevents us from entering into the kinds of mutually supportive and interdependent relationships with others and our world that are the hallmark of emotional maturity and are our truest expressions.

And the only way out of our troubles is just what Buddhism and Christianity advise. We must realize that because of our attachment (or attitude of righteousness), our conditioned and conditional ways of trying to satisfy our desires will never do the trick. Or in Christian terms, we must realize that we have to surrender to God's will for us. And the reason this way of letting go or surrender will work is because ultimately God's will is our will—immeasurable happiness, which is taught in Buddhism as the understanding that letting go of our attachments to our desires will take us down the road to the exquisite realities of higher consciousness and nirvana.

Another way for us to understand this is to apply the terms already established in the last chapter. Surrendering to God's will or detaching ourselves from our attachments to our desires means identifying with the transcendent ego, the I-viewpoint that embraces mystery or the unknowable as the central part of who we are. Our surrender, in other words, does not diminish us in any way; it increases us by establishing a living connection between who we know ourselves to be and who we will become through the guidance and support of God or Life.

Our wounded attempts to control Life will not work because who we are will always be greater than who we have been. Control will also not work because the wounding that inspires our attempts to control Life can only create crises to break us free of our self-diminishing, controlling impulse. But most of all, ego control cannot work because it does not honor the greater wisdom, heart and intelligence of the forces that seek to guide and shape us to our greatest expressions of Life's love of living.

Blame and Responsibility

Our emotional evolution is fueled in large part by the core wounding that occurs as a natural development of our growth from emotional dependence to emotional maturity, as we have seen. Yet we must also accept that emotional maturity, at least in the terms defined here, is perhaps not yet a common enough reality in our families and society for us to claim that we as a society have learned to accept the truth of who we truly are. Much of this has to do with one simple misunderstanding: we generally do not accept responsibility for our own feelings.

Yet in order to become emotionally mature, we must take responsibility for making choices that will ensure that our basic needs for safety, nurturance and guidance are met, and met in ways that do not diminish us or others. This does not mean that we must become self-sufficient, if that means that we must learn to meet our own basic needs. On the contrary, emotional maturity is not independence, but unconditional, mutually supportive interdependence. We need each other and each other's help if we ever wish to live the lives of love and creativity that are our highest potential. Love, after all, means among other things that we share the gifts of our lives with others.

Emotional maturity means that we first of all practice unconditional relationship with ourselves. We accept that no one can ever make us feel bad—because we *are* our feelings. The only way that the words or actions of another can hurt us (other than physically) is when our core wounding is activated and we somehow agree with the view of diminishment being offered us. This is a fundamental truth that rests at the heart of emotional maturity, and the proof of its validity can be found in simple examples. Untrue words, however compromising in intent, will pass right through us without evoking distress. Pain is caused by tension, and emotional pain is no exception. What we feel when we are experiencing emotional pain is connected to our core wounding, that basic hurt that comes from our living the lie of conditional worthiness. Emotional maturity means that we recognize this truth and do not assign blame for our feelings to others or to forces outside of ourselves. And if we do ever catch ourselves assigning blame to others for our feelings, emotional maturity also demands that we acknowledge this and ask for forgiveness.

The reason that having an unconditional relationship with ourselves is the foundation of emotional maturity comes from the fact that until we have established such a relationship to our personal experience, we will become unconsciously involved in emotional dependency relationships with others. Generally, we get involved in such dependency relationships because we are unconsciously brokering with others for the acceptance, approval and acknowledgment we are unable to give ourselves. For the most part, such dependency relationships mirror the areas in our life where we did not (or we perceive we did not) get our core needs met. And the fact that we are unconscious of what we are doing in emotional terms when we are involved in such conditional relationships is evidence that we have not yet taken responsibility for getting these needs met in ways that do not validate our wounded feelings of unworthiness.

Emotional maturity, in other words, means that we first of all accept ourselves to the degree that we take responsibility for any emotional feelings of distress or pain as being reflections of our core wounding—and not the fault of others. Blame, after all, goes no-where really. If we blame our parents or our culture or our boss for who we are and what we are feeling, it is not only illogical (since they in turn can blame their parents or whatever), but it is also self-limiting. Our power and our energy for personal growth and therefore our greater happiness come from standing in our absolute truth, and that truth does not recognize or accept anything but our uncondi-tional worthiness and the unconditional worthiness of others.

We must also say that emotional maturity means recognizing that whenever we are angry or upset with others or with circumstances that this, too, indicates that our core wounding of unworthiness has been activated, or triggered. Anger and its many forms are the outer-directed energies of our core wounding, and unless we take responsibility for the source of our anger we will be unable to heal, which means we will be limiting our capacity for experiencing our deepest truth. It is hopefully clear that this is not to suggest that anger or any emotion for that matter is bad and should be avoided. On the contrary, all distressing emotions are extremely valuable for their ability not only to show us the realities of our wounding, but also then to inspire our healing and lead us to increasingly greater experiences of our divinity.

That we should take responsibility for our anger and other unpleasant emotions as part of being emotionally mature does not mean that we will not at times blame others or forces outside of ourselves for what we are feeling. As emotionally mature adults we do get angry, and we do look to blame others or outside circumstances, but even in our anger or in our experiences of woundedness and blaming we are aware of what is really going on. And this means that we are then able to take full responsibility, and therefore to heal.

In regard to blame, we can recognize patterns of blaming that indicate to us the depth and character of the wounding. We tend, for example, to blame others or external forces first, and then turn the blame inward (where it also doesn't belong). This pattern of blaming corresponds to the fact that the outer-directed energy of anger is the outer layering of our wounding, and as we go deeper into our wounding we touch more of our self-diminishment.

And in terms of what our emotional evolution is all about, the touching and healing of our core wound plays a pivotal role. That is because once we have taken responsibility for the fact that our feelings are in a very direct way who we are, it becomes possible to free ourselves from the emotional entanglements and dead-ends that rob us of our life force and distract us from living the life we truly want and deserve. In other words, once we recognize the dynamics of emotional wounding, and understand them in the larger context of our emotional evolution and quest for happiness, we become empowered to consciously become engaged in the grand adventure of self-discovery, interpersonal communion, and creative expression. Until we reach such clarity, we will remain hypnotized by the dramas of blame and lack that keep us either emotionally distressed or make our lives a constant roller coaster ride between expansive highs and contractive lows.

In simpler terms, Life has a benign design, and once we have grasped that truth and chosen to cooperate with how Life guides and shapes us to our greatest happiness, our lives become infused with grace and wonder. And the key understanding is that our basic struggle is between the truth of our absolute divine worthiness and the contractive lie of our false sense of self that encourages to believe in our smallness and insignificance.

From the perspective of our wisdom traditions and teachers it seems the message is always the same—we are incredible beings with extraordinary potential for love and joyous creativity. That we have difficulty believing and understanding this truth is what holds us back perhaps more than anything else. But no one can do it for us. We must find a way to begin to let go of the fears that we are not enough or will never get enough. All that we could ever need is already within us. And once we begin to touch and accept who we truly are, the world will begin to reflect that truth back to us. That is the trick. We live in a self-reflective universe, which means that we will always attract whatever it is that we need to wake us up to our authentic being.

This idea that we will always get what we need for our emotional evolution is important to explore, especially in the context of our emotional healing. Often the notion that we live in a self-reflective universe is misunderstood to mean that if we train our minds to think only positive thoughts, or if we tell ourselves only empowering things about ourselves that we will get everything we want. While doing such things will most likely improve our lives, since we will be affirming our basic goodness, Life is not that mechanistic. And getting what we want may be a very different thing than getting what we need for our hearts to heal. As explained earlier, our desire to control Life must be surrendered if we wish to experience the truth of our being and find harmony with Life. The essential mystery of our being is a reflection of our greatness as much as it is a testament to the awesome wonder of Life itself, and this mystery must be honored and embraced for the healing of our core wounding.

Living in a self-reflective universe does mean, however, that whatever is currently present in our lives is exactly perfect and appropriate for the journey of our emotional evolution. We attract to ourselves and become emotionally involved with whatever we need not only to take us to the next level of our evolution, but also to whatever we need to help us become aware of the beauty of the moment. This is because, as stated earlier, the moment is always where it is at. Yes, Life is an ever-changing dance of moods and moments, an eternal display of impermanent forms, but the truth of each moment is absolutely eternal, and this truth is available to us with each breath we take and with each moment of our experience. And it is the simple recognition that each moment is an opportunity for us to know and feel the truth of our being that does more to inspire us and our healing than anything else.

Of course accepting that the bad relationship we are in or the grief we are feeling for the passing of a loved one is what we need for our healing and for realizing the truth of our divinity is quite a challenge. It requires not only that we surrender our fears of lack, but also that we learn to honor whatever feelings we are experiencing as being the best vehicle for the evolution of our hearts and minds. This is because emotional experience is the way that our hearts evolve, and therefore how we grow in love and understanding. And when we can apply our understandings of core emotional wounding, and accept at least the possibility that what we are feeling is our own wounding, then we will be taking conscious steps toward our healing—and these steps will be responded to by the self-reflective nature of Life that seeks to support and guide us in every moment to our highest truth.

So whatever our emotional experience happens to be, it is our guide. And in this respect there is no better guide than human relationship. Human relationship is where our emotional evolution journey begins, and it in effect remains the context and focus of nearly all of our emotional energy throughout our lives. For this reason, it is essential that we learn the dynamics of human relationship so that we may wisely choose not only the kinds of relationships that will serve us and others best, but also so that we can understand how to best work with the interplay of emotional wounding that is a part of all relationships. For this reason, defensive patterns, projection, triggering and relationship mirroring are concepts that will be explored in detail later in the book. First, however, we must be clear about how emotion and mind function together in our sense-making, and for this we will turn to how our ideas and assumptions about Life are emotionally based.

Faces of the Creator

As we look around the world or even our own neighborhoods, we quickly come to see that our traditions and cultures have come to understand and to represent our human perceptions of Life's Creator in a rich variety of ways. Even those who imagine that our universe is truly without a conscious creating force or intelligence, frame their perceptions is a multitude of ways that reflect their deepest assumptions and beliefs about Life's design and order. In fact all ideas we have about the nature and intention of a Creator or of Life involve the interplay between the three modes of our human experience: the physical, the emotional, and the imaginative. And since these ideas about a Creator or Life itself are so fundamental, and inform or affect all of our choices, we would be wise not only to examine them, but also to understand how our emotions and especially how our emotional wounding play a role in these basic beliefs.

At the outset, we must first of all concede that just as we cannot fully imagine the extent of our own being because our very nature is transcendent, we are of course not able to fully conceive or imagine our Creator or even the design of Life. This is the ultimate challenge in religious, spiritual or mystical thought: trying to conceive of something that must at some level be beyond our conceptual ability. But in experiential terms, when contemplating Life or Life's Creator it perhaps doesn't matter as much what name we have—Creator, God, Allah, Great Spirit, All That Is, Goddess, I Am, All Love Beingness—because the name is a form through which we access the experience. Some traditions, in fact, shroud the symbol or name of the Creator in mystery, paradox, or even silence as a way to signify how limited our conceptions must be.

All of this actually supports the idea that truth is primarily emotional (as in the experience of unconditional love), and alerts us to the greater limitations of our mind experience when it comes to the experience of truth. Heart, or emotion, is after all the gate of transcendence, not mind. At the same time, however, it is important for us to realize that whatever name we use to signify Life's Creator for ourselves, this name or symbol reflects a conception that underlies all experiences of self. And this is the point; these fundamental beliefs or assumptions about Life and a Creator will reveal much about ourselves, and much about the connection between mind and emotion.

Naturally, much of how we conceive of Life or Life's Creator is handed down to us through our families and cultures, and for this reason we do not always look very closely. Often in fact these fundamental ideas and beliefs are so taken for granted that they are virtually invisible, scribbled deep into the patterns of our identity. Yet because they are so vitally a part of how we see ourselves and the world they are quite valuable for how they affect the choices we are making. If, for example, we perceive of Life's Creator as a paternal authority, this will have emotional effects, as will a belief that our Creator is frivolous and absent-minded. The point of course is that our ideas about such things are bound to contain some elements of emotional projection. In other words, we place into our ideas that which we desire to be true, or fear to be true. In either case, our emotional reality will become a part of whatever ideas we have about the nature and intentions of our Creator, and this can have important consequences.

One interesting way to shake out projections regarding the faces of Life's Creator is to take a small step back from our conceptions and pay attention to what metaphors or models we find to fit our sense of our personal relationship to our Creator and to Life. This can even be quite fun as we learn to distinguish the aspects of ourselves doing the projecting.

1. A Family. In this model the Creator is one or somehow both of the parents.

2. A Science Project. No Creator, just lots of random forces that miraculously created the conditions for Life from a teaspoon or so of heavy matter. Essentially, we got luckier than the biggest lottery winner ever.

3. A Garden or Playground. In this story we can do whatever we choose, and all will be provided as long as we are having fun.

4. A School. Here the Creator is either a cranky taskmaster or a kind teacher showing us how to start vegetables in milk cartons.

5. A Battlefield. In this drama the armies of Good face down the forces of Evil. We're just waiting for the Good side's secret weapon to be unleashed.

6. A Movie. This version has all of us as projections, holographic or otherwise, and the bad actors seem to get all the best parts.

7.   Heaven's Boring. This inventive variation on the Movie model has all of us as angels who sneak away for Star Trek style holodeck role playing. As temporary amnesiacs we think it's all for real and manage to scare the living beejeezus out of ourselves.

8.   The Exploding God. Apparently the Big Bang blew God into infinite pieces, and we've all got a piece. Fortunately, the in-breath will put us back together. Humpty Dumpty with a twist.

In fact all of these models, together with others, highlight characteristics of Life that somehow seem to reflect how we make sense of what we experience in our lives. The point in taking a lighthearted look at them is to provide some critical distance so that we might begin to see how emotionally attached we may be to the more serious versions of these world views. In any case, we need to understand how our most serious beliefs about who we are, and therefore about Life and Life's Creator, are certain to be somehow involved in our essential wounding. Even though we may not be able to imagine or fully understand how Life works or what God's true nature may be, we will be able to feel and experience how the healing of our emotional wounding will open us to greater experiences of love and joyous creating. And it is the heart, not the mind that ultimately determines how happy we are.

One final point before we have more fun and look closely at *The Wizard of Oz* as a model for a transcendent journey: our ideas will always contain our emotional wounding and other emotional realities. This is because the mind must always incorporate our emotional experience in its imaginings. That is why it can be so difficult to emotionally heal through understanding our traumas. It's as if the wounding is in the actual walls of the stories or explanations we use to understand. Or, to use the terminology we have been using, our emotional wounding is throughout our experience, and this includes the physical as well as the emotional and imaginative modes of our experience. And, as we shall see, true healing requires that we learn to heal and unwind our wounding through all three modes of human experience.

Chapter Two Main Points

1.   Unconditional love is the measure or standard for personal truth. Practical Application: Understanding that emotion is the path to personal truth motivates us to understand emotional dynamics.

2.   The human emotional journey begins with emotional dependency and idealization. Practical Application: Once aware of our emotional inheritance, we can begin to more readily identify the authentic self that transcends (goes beyond and includes) our inheritance.

3.   Our essential evolutionary dynamic is created from the tension between the inner knowingness of our absolute worthiness and the conditionality reflected back to us from our families and cultures. Practical Application: Understanding that this dynamic is an essential part of Life's design allows us to more consciously transform our conditional identity.

4.   Emotional maturity requires that we learn to be responsible for making choices that ensure that our needs for safety, nurturance and guidance are met. Practical Application: When we learn to identify our core needs we can take steps to make sure they are unconditionally met.

5.   Human lives are framed and fashioned by the suffering that results from the misguided belief that we know what we truly want and what is best for us. Practical Application: Surrendering the desires of the conditional self begins to reveal our authentic identity.

6.   Emotional wounding is the painful tension that results from accepting any conditional identity over the unconditional identity of our absolute divinity. Practical Application: We can learn to undo the compartmentalization that has us creating conditional relationships with others in order to find approval.

7.   The only emotional wound is the pain we feel when we are not recognized (even by ourselves) for the truth of our unconditional worthiness. Practical Application: Understanding that anger and self-diminishment are reflections of our inner sense of not being recognized as worthy allows us to stop blaming others for our feelings so that we can heal and evolve toward emotional enlightenment.

8.   The emotional dynamics of our core wounding are unavoidable, and they always center around feelings of lack. Practical Application: When we realize that we are of course already good enough we can begin to heal our core wounding and create more room for our authentic being to emerge.

9.   Becoming emotionally mature means taking responsibility for our feelings. Practical Application: We are freed by the truth that no one can make us feel bad—the fact that we are the only ones who can make us feel bad motivates and empowers us to heal.

10. Emotion, not mind, is the gate of transcendence. Practical Application: Examining our core beliefs for their emotional content and degree of emotional maturity will bring growth.

Exercise for Experiential Understanding

This exercise can have many outcomes. It may make you aware of unconscious ideas you have about Life and Life's Creator and open the way for deeper understanding and new growth. You may discover strong feelings you were unaware of, and their expression may free you in unexpected ways. It is also possible that you will tap into a well of joy and vitality that will inspire and energize you. You will need pen and paper.

Write a poem, letter or song directly addressed to Life's Creator. In your creative writing describe Life's Creator using as many details as you can. As much as possible, tap into and express any emotions you may feel, whether you consider them appropriate or not. If you find that you are not making any progress on a poem or song, try writing a personal letter first. For models and inspiration, you may wish to consult religious writings from your own religion or others. If this seems too serious, try a humorous or lighthearted approach.

Make sure you take the time necessary to review your work over the course of at least several days so that you may deepen your ideas. When you feel that you have finished your piece, you may wish to share it with loved ones.

Questions for Contemplation

What gets me angry? What does this tell me about my underlying emotional wounding? What are my patterns for blame when I get angry? Whom do I blame more—myself, others or Life? What can I do to begin to heal, to become whole?

Notes:

The Adventure of Self-Discovery

Life at its best is an adventure, first of all of self-discovery, and then of exuberant creativity. The thrill of the adventure comes in large part from the many surprises that await us at every turn in the road. But these surprises can emotionally upend us if we aren't aware that each obstacle or challenge we face asks the same question: Who are You? And it depends upon how deeply we are buried in the lies of our unknowing and unworthiness whether we can rise to these challenges and stand or even dance in our deepest truth.

The process of self-discovery that marks the first part of our journey on the way to emotional maturity can be undeniably treacherous. Life demands that we learn not only to recognize that we are being asked the same question over and over again, but that we gain the confidence and trust to answer without hesitation. And once we can do that, once we can clearly state who we truly are as our answer to Life's persistent challenges, deep healing and true connection to others and to Life begins.

But what is the nature and purpose of such healing? If we manage to find that gentle stillpoint in ourselves where we can unflinchingly stand our ground to the onslaught of fears and the temptations to doubt ourselves, shouldn't that be it? Haven't we finished the quest and found our bliss? After all, that's what seems to happen in our movies and in our hero/heroine stories. Our happy endings are about happily ever after, not happiness *and* healing; they're about riding off into the sunset or leaving for the honeymoon or retiring to an island in the sun with a cell phone and a Swiss bank account.

It's interesting that our popular stories leave off right where it would be nice to have some insight into what happens once you've made it, once you've managed to really get who you are. Perhaps it's simply that the self-discovery part of the journey is more familiar, and that we've not yet really learned how to do the next bit. Or maybe we imagine happiness to be boring, and think that once you've gotten the girl or wedded the guy or struck it rich or escaped from your cruelest prison that you've reached your highest peak. But as fun and adventurous as self-discovery is, the potential is for things to really just get better—and more exciting—from there.

Life's adventure continues after true self-discovery, after uncon-ditional self-acceptance and emotional maturity, and it continues to become better and better. That's because the healing that follows self-discovery (and is such an integral part of emotional maturity) allows us to really develop or perhaps even uncover for the first time our life's creative purpose. Maybe this is why Life is so persistent in the first place: the really good stuff can only come out once we've recognized ourselves as absolutely worthy of it.

It's no great mystery that our greatest happiness comes from a life full of love and creative expression. Life, after all, is itself all about love and the love of creating new forms to be loved. What seems to be less understood, however, is that the full flowering of love can only happen in our lives once we have claimed and experienced our own divinity. This is true because we can only recognize the abso-lute worthiness and goodness of others to the degree that we have discovered ourselves to be unconditionally worthy of all that will make our lives truly wonderful.

Moreover, our highest creative expression will only come about once we have healed ourselves of the self-destructive attitudes and behaviors borne of our identification with our conditional egos. In other words, the healing process is actually the formation of our highest creative self. We are of course creative throughout our lives, often incredibly so, but not to our potential. And that creative potential can only be unlocked and fueled by the unconditional love made possible by our unconditional self-approval. In ideal terms, therefore, the adventure of becoming is an unfolding (and often interwoven) process of self-discovery, healing, and creative expression.

The steps or stages of that process will be more or less the outline for the remainder of the book. This chapter will look closely at *The Wizard of Oz* as a model for the transformational process of self-discovery. The following chapters will focus on emotional healing, or the peeling back of the layers of self-negation that armor the human heart. From there we will explore issues of work and creativity, with an emphasis on learning to create and live the life of your highest creative expression.

Collective Story Making

Stories, as we all learn in school, can be full of all kinds of relatively hidden symbols for the universal elements of love, truth and beauty—in a seemingly infinite display of form. What may seem on the surface to be fairly ordinary, can be revealed to be just the top waves in an ocean full of powerful, often predictable currents and tides. So it is also with the stories of our lives. We may have come to see the surface of our lives as rather commonplace or ordinary, but the deeper truth is much different. For the most part we simply do not take the time to feel or become aware of all that is going on beneath the surface.

This idea that a great deal of our being exists somehow outside of our conscious experience, and that getting in touch with the under-currents and forces that influence us will lead to greater well being is of course not new. Religions and psychology are in fact reliant on the fact that we have access within us to what we need for our heal-ing and redemption. The stories of our lives, therefore, are where we should turn for the clues and insights into what is going on outside of our conscious awareness.

The psychologist Carl Jung's idea of the collective unconscious adds another interesting dimension to looking at our life stories. This shared pool of human experience that links each of us with the ex-periences of our ancestors and indeed all humanity through common symbols, or archetypes, is useful for looking at how our personal ex-perience is linked to all of human experience. But whatever one makes of Jung's concept, it and similar ideas underscore and point to an important aspect of Life's design. We are never alone, and our journeys and stories rely on and are deeply involved in the journeys and stories of others.

Life is the Grand Storymaker, with all of us playing roles in the life stories of others as well as in the overall collective stories of our families, friends, cultures and even in the collective story of human-ity. Each of us, and each of our stories, however, is decidedly unique. We may share the same basic structures, symbols and archetypes for our stories and personal sense-making, but each story is a unique mixture or constellation of story elements. This holds true also for our communal or collective stories. And no matter the scope or size of a story, what unifies and remains constant is the impulse toward transcendence and greater meaning.

Stories, in other words, are always about personal experiences of growth and transformation, even when the story is a shared or col-lective one. The story of human history, for example, may be the chronicle and record of human activity and desire, but it only truly becomes significant when the story or an aspect of the story personally inspires someone and gives that individual's life greater meaning.

Story, as the language of Life's creation, delights, moves, instructs and inspires us in our experiences of transcendence. It is not surprising, therefore, that our most prized shared stories are rich in dramatic tension, wisdom, humor and heart, for these are the stories that speak to our individual journeys of transcendence. And because the stories of our individual journeys use shared basic elements for meaning, and follow the same metaphoric or associative logic in design, we can learn much about ourselves and the ways of Life when we look closely at a collective story's symbolic or archetypal content.

This is of course what we do when we learn and study religious and moral stories, but the opportunity for personal growth is possible when any story touches our hearts. Classical and popular myths, for example, as stories inspired and shaped over time by the collective truths of human experience, are quite rich in symbols that resonate within us, and we are wise to pay close attention to all symbols and stories that move us.

In this regard the stories of our dreams are especially potent, for they contain symbols and narratives that directly connect us to our deeper experiences and offer us clues and signposts for transcendence. The difficulty in learning and understanding the language of dreams may often pose something of a challenge, but as soon as we begin to understand the associative nature of dreams and look for the emotional content of dream stories and symbols, the more accessible our dream content becomes.

Dreams, in other words, are not intentionally mysterious—although dream meanings can be elusive and even vexing. Part of the reason for this comes from our efforts to try and understand dreams only in terms of our waking, conscious awareness. Dreams display both conscious and unconscious elements of our overall being, and it is therefore necessary to bridge both worlds in order to make sense of our dreams. That means we must know that the common links between waking reality and dream reality are emotional experience and associative or metaphoric sense-making. We should also realize that dreams offer us access to dimensions of ourselves that lie outside the selective conscious mind, and dreams are therefore a wonderful place to begin to sort out our anxieties and woundedness for the purposes of self-discovery and healing. This requires that we learn to make sense of dream language and dream logic, which means we must also understand the fundamentals of symbols and symbol making in stories.

Perhaps the most important thing to understand for making sense of the symbolic language of dreams is that dream symbols are both created and revealed. In other words, in our dreams we create symbols out of our individual experiences, and we also encounter archetypes, or symbols for forces that already exist, even if only in potential. We may, for example, use familiar objects or persons from our daily lives for our dream making, and simultaneously available to us are the greater symbols of all human experience such as the elements and forms of nature. Both created and revealed symbols, however, always relate somehow to our personal story when they are part of a dream, and it is how we put these symbols together when we are in our conscious waking state that determines how well we understand and can act upon the stories of our dreams.

In order to do this, we must learn to effectively use the languages of waking reality and of dream logic, which for the most part involves applying associative reasoning to the emotional content of a dream. In other words, although we cannot fully separate the form from the experience, in both waking and dream states it is the experience and not necessarily the form of the experience that creates meaning.

To Oz and Back

As stories that are rich in archetypes and symbols, myths teach us a great deal about the human experience. Like any story, however, a myth is only as powerful as the feelings and thoughts it inspires, and for this reason myths must be renewed and new myths must be created by a culture in order to move, guide and delight the people living in a specific era and community. In ancient oral traditions (and in some modern ones the practice continues) this was done by storytellers who learned the community's stories and told them, with embellishments meant to be improvements for reaching a contemporary audience, often at community gatherings.

The best of such stories spoke to a listener's unconscious as well as conscious understanding, so that while the listener didn't always grasp the story on a literal level, the archetypes and elements within the story stirred resonances between personal and universal human experience. Similar storytelling occurs today, and our most popular medium for such storytelling has become film. This brings of course a whole new set of storytelling and story-making considerations to our myth making, but at root the same potential for powerful myths to inspire our transcendence is alive and well.

Evidence of the vitality of our storytelling through film is abundant, but what is often missing in our collective stories is the information regarding transcendence that was passed down in figurative (non-literal, or metaphoric) form in the oral traditions. From the perspective of emotional evolution, our films often lack the positive allegorical and symbolic dimensions that are needed to speak to us and inform us about how to satisfy our thirst and need for transcendence.

Occasionally, of course, films are made that wonderfully satisfy the requirements for an honest-to-goodness myth of transcendence, but as we are not in the general habit of watching films repeatedly in the way that myths in oral traditions were repeated with regularity, these films do not have the opportunity to work on us from within to the same degree. We do not, in other words, allow such a film's archetypal content and dream logic to be woven into the fabric of our individual journeys.

A notable exception to this has been the film *The Wizard of Oz,* which despite its reputation as a frivolous fantasy for children, has all the elements for a genuine myth of transcendence. This is shown by the fact that the film's subject matter is positive personal growth; that it is seen repeatedly by a large, intergenerational population; and that it contains effective symbolism to reflect the trials of a hero-ine seeking to identify with her transcendent self and discovery her true identity. The film is also a lot of fun.

For these reasons, it's useful to take a close look at *The Wizard of Oz* for instruction in the ways of story, dream logic and authentic self-discovery. (You may wish to watch this film again, either before or immediately following your reading of this chapter.) Dorothy Gale's journey is a story of personal quest, and as such it speaks directly to the myth maker and seeker in all of us. Dorothy's fantastic journey to Oz is in fact full of archetypal symbolism and serves as a wonder-ful primer for dream language and logic, and for the personal growth that accompanies transcendence.

As a story relating to the collective unconscious it is also quite interesting, especially when we consider the context of the film's creation as part of the overall story. What comes off on screen as relatively seamless belies the actual process of the production, which saw at least four directors, many writers, and the usual casting and production intrigues. When the addition of the extremely talented Judy Garland (as Dorothy) and her own personal struggles is made, the fact that the film was ever completed is in itself something of a miracle. Yet this is precisely the magic of the transcendent journey.

In critical interpretations of *The Wizard of Oz*, much has been made of the relationship between the film and the original book, an allegory for children by L. Frank Baum called *The Wonderful Wizard of Oz*, and even many of those who have treated the film on its own have tended to see it as a brand of Hollywood escapism awkwardly laced with moral messages for would-be rebels and dissenters. What seems lacking in such interpretation, however, is an appreciation for how the film has functioned as a cultural myth and the degree to which it mirrors the process of transcendence.

Millions of people have watched this film, some of them count-less times, and many can recite from it and its many songs at the slightest prodding. (It is, by the way, the Lollipop Guild, not the Lollipop Kids.) For others, the film evokes memories of childhood fears—especially the dark scenes at the castle with the Wicked Witch's flying monkeys. Yet perhaps most of all, the film is valuable for its spirit. This spirit is one of the dreamworld, where time and space become jumbled and blended with inner wisdom and an op-portunity to face our demons—which turn out to be aspects of ourselves. And in all of this there is the presence of the enigmatic workings of dream logic, which forces itself onto the stage and shows itself to be the equal of the usual linear, cause and effect logic associ-ated with waking consciousness.

In regard to the film's symbolism, it is remarkable that although much of it is deliberate, coming as it does from Baum's allegory, other aspects of the symbolism which are less obvious emerge from storytelling traditions and perspectives as diverse as Native Ameri-can mythology and Germanic folklore. This is the result of the story's intentional treatment of themes that lie at the heart of human ex-perience—the struggle for identity and personal empowerment.

The appearance of such unexpected symbolism is not accidental; archetypes and symbols of the collective unconscious work deeply, and most often out of conscious awareness. From this perspective it is less surprising but nevertheless wondrous that Dorothy's journey mirrors the characteristics of a shamanic journey. Dorothy, as a shaman or healer, travels to another dimension of reality, where she directly confronts the fearful elements of an identity crisis precipitated by her steps over the threshold lying between girlhood and empowerment. On her journey she searches within herself for what is needed for the healing, and aided by her inner guides and wisdom Dorothy uncovers truths that will serve to continually remind her of her real identity as a shaman or wizard. The power of myth is evoked when through her journey Dorothy unconsciously reminds us of our own innate goodness and positive wizardry. The fact that we are dealing with a potent myth will also require that we pay attention to the dream logic and archetypal symbolism that finds its way to the story's surface.

A Witch in the House

Dorothy's confrontation with Miss Gulch in the opening scenes of the movie becomes the catalyst for the greater identity crisis that has been brewing already for some time. Nobody in Dorothy's extended family will listen to her about her problems with Miss Gulch, and Aunt Em gives the worn adult response to Dorothy's "over-emotional" nature when she comments that Dorothy always gets herself "in a fret over nothing." But for Dorothy this is clearly a true emergency, and when Miss Gulch is granted the communal authority to do away with Dorothy's dog, Toto, Dorothy rebels against such injustice to the full extent of her voice.

Appeals to her Aunt Em and Uncle Henry, however, are useless, and Dorothy simply can't believe or accept their impotence. In terms of her emotional evolution, her idealization of her step-parents faces a real test that for the sake of Dorothy's continued self-emergence will have to fail. Only minutes before Miss Gulch's arrival at the farm Dorothy had sung her anthem of liberation, "Somewhere Over the Rainbow," and when Toto easily escapes the clutches of Miss Gulch they run away—hopefully to the place of no troubles where "the dreams you dare to dream really do come true" and where you and all others are seen for who they truly are.

It is clear from this opening scene that Dorothy chooses a path of transcendence by consciously standing up for her truth. Had she mutely accepted the injustice of the situation it would have set an inhibiting precedent, for transcendent growth is dependent upon how fully we actualize our inner identity in the outside world. But Dorothy *Gale* was a storm waiting to happen, as we soon see. Not only does she allow the anger and emotional pain of her core wounding to be expressed, but in doing so she also brands the powerful Miss Gulch a witch. This turns out to be significant for the dream-state portion of the film, where Gulch in fact becomes the Wicked Witch of the East.

In this regard it is interesting that *gulch* is a word whose Germanic origin means to swallow greedily, which fits Miss Gulch's strident possessiveness (she owns half the county) quite well. That witches then play such an important role in Dorothy's journey of self-healing, where all characters are partial reflections of herself, emphasizes how it is through the magic of transcendence that what has appeared to be evil and ugly is revealed to be divine.

Dorothy runs away from those who love her because in the clarity brought on by a crisis she sees that things are not as she had believed. Aunt Em and Uncle Henry are shown to be powerless exactly when it counts the most—which leads to Dorothy's important intuitive insight that she isn't one of her own family. Family and community, in fact, are important issues of Dorothy's identity crisis, and it is significant that in the story she is an orphan. This reflects the apparent condition of all seekers, for as much as we are connected to our families, it seems also true that we come through and not from them. Our families and connections are only one aspect of our greater identities, and in our journey of transcendence we all face the fears and realities of this kind of orphanhood.

In the Oz story, Dorothy the actual orphan lives with her aunt and uncle on their Kansas farm, where she adopts as part of her extended family the three farmhands whose reflections later become Scarecrow, Tin Man and Lion. It is symbolically significant that the entire crisis revolves around Toto, the dog Dorothy unconditionally loves and protects. Her identity, her unconscious knowing of her transcendent self, is reliant upon Toto, so when Toto is threatened so is she. The name Toto supports this idea, as in the Latin phrase *in toto*, meaning 'as a whole.' Dorothy's wholeness, her divinity and absolute worthiness are her essential truth.

Applying Native American perspectives is also interesting in this story, and they are justified because they are part of the lore and archetypal heritage of Dorothy's land. And in this case, a Native American perspective yields even further significance to Toto's name. On the one hand, the Algonquin word *totem* refers to an animal or natural object taken as the symbol of a family or clan and is therefore closely linked to personal identity. In addition, the traditional medicine or power of the dog is the teaching of loyalty, which in Dorothy's case refers to her need to be true to her divine self, or Self.

Dorothy's actual journey begins when she leaves the farm, running away with Toto into the unknown. Immediately she meets her first guide, Professor Marvel. That he is a charlatan doesn't matter;

for Dorothy his being and words take on mystical qualities because he, from her naïve perspective, seems worldly and wise. His advice to her to return home is both practical and inspired: it is only by returning home to her true, unconditionally worthy Self that Dorothy can find what she is looking for. He also performs the task of getting Dorothy to see that she has brought her troubles upon herself. As Dorothy admits, she could have prevented Toto from chasing Gulch's cat in the first place, and the pain she feels at having caused Aunt Em's heartache by running away was equally avoidable.

This realization reveals that the nature of this crisis is to facilitate her emotional development from dependence to emotional maturity. As an adolescent Dorothy is caught between the worlds of childhood and adulthood, which means she must undergo the often painful lessons that go along with self responsibility. But her true test is whether or not she can manage to keep her heart open when faced with the apparent injustices of the world, for in one sense her indignation and desire to flee are reflections of the insecurities she feels in the face of her stepping into the adult world. Her anger and willingness to leave it all behind her show that she is very much a captive of the conditional world of blame, a world that exists solely in her own wounded heart.

Over the Rainbow

By the time Dorothy and Toto get back to the farm, everyone has already taken shelter below ground, and they seek protection from the storm in the house. The problem, of course, is that the twister can't be escaped. Dorothy has let go of her old identity, symbolized by the house, her home, and the storm that ensues is Dorothy's own doing. That a window (representing her self view or outlook) then knocks her unconscious further emphasizes this dimension of her identity crisis. On the transcendent journey, unconscious aspects of the self become conscious, and now that Dorothy has fully let go of conscious control, everything that she will need to complete her current growth process will naturally come her way. This is not to say that she must abandon her conscious mind; it is only that she has surrendered its dominance to the greater wisdom of her entire being.

When Dorothy lands in Munchkinland, she steps into the technicolor world of a waking dream state. As a shaman she has journeyed deep into her being in order to take back whatever wisdom she will need to heal herself. It is not surprising in this context that she lands in a world populated by eternal children, for it is the transformation from child to adult that she must make. In Munchkinland she is honored for having killed the Wicked Witch of the East, known of course in Dorothy's waking consciousness as Miss Gulch. Naturally Dorothy expresses some regret at having killed the witch, explaining to all that it was merely a coincidence, but since this witch has reportedly tormented the inhabitants of Munchkinland she is nonetheless a heroine.

It is here in Munchkinland that the whole issue of Dorothy's empowerment first takes stage. Glinda, the Good Witch of the North who magically appears out of a glowing orb, immediately phrases the moral dimension of Dorothy's new status when she asks, "Are you a good witch or a bad witch?" That there even existed such a thing as a good witch was news to Dorothy before she met Glinda, but Dorothy is already quite sure that she is one of the good witches.

At this point, right on cue, the Wicked Witch of the West rides in to avenge the death of her sister, and Dorothy discovers she now has a mortal enemy. From the perspective of her self-discovery, it appears that Dorothy's empowerment will have to be earned before she can fully step into it. Glinda, as an alert guide, presses this issue by reminding the Witch of the magical ruby slippers, but then right before the Witch can get to them Glinda transfers the slippers to Dorothy's feet. This not only strengthens the notion that all of the characters in the lucid dream are dimensions of Dorothy, but it also ensures the necessary enmity between Dorothy and her next inner challenge for growth and transcendence, the Wicked Witch of the West.

Clarissa Pinkola Estés in her book *Women Who Run With the Wolves* explains the significance of red shoes in fairy tales by referring to them as a psychological metaphor for the freedom and mobility to live a vibrant life. In Dorothy's case Glinda informs her that these shoes will protect her on her quest to return home, and they are in effect Dorothy's broom— both a symbol of power and a means of transportation. But first she must learn to use her new shoes, which means she must make the trip on foot to Oz to see the Wizard, who will certainly be able to help her get back to Kansas. The danger of the situation, however, is clear. The Wicked Witch of the West has vowed revenge, and even Glinda has admitted that Dorothy is up against a formidable foe.

Off to See the Wizard

The road to the Emerald City of course begins in Munchkinland, and Dorothy sets out right away— her only instruction from Glinda being to follow the yellow brick road. But she has her ruby red shoes for protection, and along the way she is joined by three traveling companions who become convinced that the Wizard can also solve their problems. What is immediately interesting about Scarecrow, Tin Man and Lion is that they, like Dorothy, are incomplete. In fact, they all feel themselves to be a failure in some sense because of what appears to be lacking. The Scarecrow lacks a brain; the Tin Man's tinsmith forgot to give him a heart; and the Lion, though king of the beasts, is a coward. All, including Dorothy, are seeking empowerment, and with Dorothy's encouragement they accept that the wonderful Wizard of Oz will certainly be able to make them whole.

That a sense of lack or incompleteness is what propels all four of them is archetypal. The perception of not having or not being enough is the driving force of our search for ourselves, and we set out on the adventure of self-discovery thinking we can find what we need somewhere else or from someone else. This, however, is Life's plan for us, for the challenges and obstacles we attract in our searching serve to draw us out of ourselves so that we may one day understand that the source of our troubles, as well as the source of our redemption, lies within.

Dorothy's situation, however, is clearly different from the others because her predicament includes all of their woes. Her search for a way back home is a desire to know the original state of her eternal, unconditional being, and in order to do so she must connect and integrate with her transcendent self. This will require all of the qualities her friends find lacking in themselves: intelligence, love and courage. Of course it is evident in the movie that these qualities are already a part of the characters of her companions; it is simply that they do not see themselves. Scarecrow's intelligence is obvious from the start, not only in the fact that he can speak, but in how he outwits the apple tree in order to get some fruit for himself and Dorothy. Tin Man's heart is open and functioning, and his dance for joy when he has been released from the constriction of rusting is ample evidence of this.

Lion is apparently the most needy, and that is due to his extreme emotional sensitivity and his fear of that sensitivity. Courage, as a quality of heart, is perhaps the most difficult but necessary quality for those on a conscious path of transcendence. The word courage, in fact, comes from the Latin word for heart, and its meaning can perhaps best be paraphrased as wisdom of the heart, for true courage is the heartfelt understanding that our greatest strength as beings of joy is our ability to open our hearts without fear. This is the greatest and most difficult of Life's lessons, and the fact that Lion even consents to face his fears is ample proof of his innate courage.

The three friends Dorothy makes along the way are in a very real sense her spiritual guides and protectors. It is interesting from an esoteric perspective that her friends represent the animal (Lion), vegetable (Scarecrow) and mineral (Tin Man) realms of being. As a member of the human realm Dorothy contains all of these aspects within herself, so it is in a very direct sense that the guidance she receives comes from her inner being. And she will certainly need this guidance to confront her larger demons as she moves toward greater wholeness. To an extent she can rely on the strength of her innate goodness, represented by Glinda, to get her through the minor trials of her life (as when Glinda let snow fall to overcome the poison poppy field the Wicked Witch placed in Dorothy's path), but when the time comes for her to really step into herself she will have to consciously face her greatest fears.

The Great and Powerful Oz

Once they have been admitted into the Emerald City on the testimonial of the ruby slippers, Dorothy and her friends believe all their problems are over. They celebrate and prepare for an audience with the Wizard by getting groomed and fussed over by the joyous inhabitants of Oz. It does in fact seem that they have overcome many trials to get there, and the city of Oz is as wonderful as they had dreamed. It resembles that "somewhere over the rainbow" Dorothy had sung about—where only good things happen and everyone cooperates and is happy all the time. But then, just when things appear brightest, the Wicked Witch of the West shows up and frightens the citizens of Oz by skywriting the message that Dorothy should surrender.

That the Wicked Witch of the West demands that Dorothy surrender is inspired, and reveals the deeper forces of myth breaking through to the surface of the narrative. Dorothy will of course have to surrender her false sense of self, which includes her fears and her feelings of incompleteness and unworthiness, in order to connect with the truth of her divine identity. As detailed in the last chapter, this means we must surrender our attachment to our desires, which requires that we must also surrender our efforts to control Life because our conceptions of who we may become are limited by our emotional wounding. That it is the Witch who demands Dorothy surrender is further evidence of this, for the Witch is a reflection of Dorothy's core wounding.

At this point it is also important to note that there are often stages in the transcendent process that offer rest and give the seeker a much needed sense of accomplishment and confidence. These periods, however, occasionally provide refreshment right before the greatest challenges—which is another reason why it is wise to replenish ourselves through rest and celebration when the occasion arises. And using once again the symbol of a house to stand for identity, it is clearly true that celebration is in order—Dorothy's sense of self has already expanded considerably. Oz, as a self-contained palace, is vastly larger and more secure than the house in which she traveled to Munchkinland. Yet there are still a few problems to be worked out— not least of which is a pesky witch insistent upon getting even. Trusting in the magic and wonderful works of the Wizard, however, Dorothy and her companions are at first not at all worried.

Yet getting in to see the Wizard turns out to be a problem in itself, solved only by the palace guard's effusive empathy for Dorothy and her story. And once the four seekers are actually granted an audience, things do not get easier. Oz of course knows in advance why they have come to him, and he succeeds in frightening Dorothy's friends. But Dorothy herself is not shaken, and she displays her characteristic streak of outspokenness at their mistreatment by the Wizard. Her courage and sense of purpose save the day, or at least provide a temporary stay. The Wizard gives in by promising to grant their wishes in exchange for the broomstick of the Wicked Witch, an extremely challenging task that is in essence asking them to do away with the Witch. However, since Dorothy in a larger sense is of course most interested in being free of her woundedness, such a request was inevitable, and the broom works as a definite symbol of her potential power and liberation.

Ding, Dong the Wicked Witch is Dead

With no alternative, Dorothy and the others gladly take on the task and proceed to the darkness of the Enchanted Forest. A dark forest is traditionally seen as a symbol of what is fearful in the unconscious, and here they are indeed easy prey for the Witch. Dorothy and Toto are immediately apprehended by the flying monkeys, and they are taken away to the dark castle, Oz's shadow city. Considered nothing more than a nuisance by the Witch, Dorothy's guides are left alone though badly shaken by the attack of the Witch's flying troops.

Back in the castle, the Witch tries to exchange Toto for the ruby slippers, to which Dorothy might have been tempted to agree, but the magic of the slippers necessitates that the wearer die before they can be taken off. The Witch gleefully gives Dorothy an hour to live, but not before Toto, quite adept at outsmarting those who underestimate him, makes a run for it and escapes. Dorothy shouts encouragement after Toto and is emotionally strengthened by this important victory.

These events all happen rather quickly, and it becomes increasingly clear that a confrontation between Dorothy and her shadow figure is unavoidable. And on the surface, things do not look good for Dorothy, who has apparently been rendered completely powerless, trapped without her dog or her guides to protect her. Significantly, this is exactly what she most fears, and as she watches the hourglass she calls out in vain to Auntie Em. This is a moment of reckoning, where Life has conspired with her own choices to create a situation where she will be forced to answer the persistent question of who she truly is while under the potent stresses of fear and doubt.

Yet it is only Dorothy's conscious ego mind that perceives itself alone and separated, and this perception is the source of her woundedness. In reality her inner strengths have been marshalled together and are preparing for an all-out confrontation with the Witch. In this context it is interesting that Toto, Dorothy's symbol of spiritual wholeness, is the agent that shows the others the way to the dark castle. Once there, they are ambushed by three of the Witch's guard, but they quickly turn the tables and proceed inside by disguising themselves with the guards' uniforms.

In the final scene with the Wicked Witch of the West it is important to note that like her sister, the Wicked Witch of the East, she was killed by accident. Of course this is done on one level to preserve Dorothy's innocence in the eyes of the audience, who identifies with Dorothy and her plight, but there are other reasons as well. First of all, as reflections or aspects of Dorothy's transcendent self these shadow figures cannot be killed; they can be either repressed or integrated in some fashion into the whole of her being. This is shown by the fact that in both cases during the movie there is no body that remains after the accident. The first witch simply shrivels up and is sucked under the house that landed on her, and the Wicked Witch of the West melts away when doused by water (the element of emotion) meant to put out Scarecrow. These disappearing bodies signify that Dorothy has successfully met her inner demons and integrated them into her expanding identity.

The idea of accidents killing the Witches is also significant when one considers that in the context of a dream state there are no coincidences. Everything happens right on time because the conscious conception of orderly time is simply used as a convention or device in dreaming. The dreamer can mix and match events and people regardless of chronology, for in the dream world what matters is not just the logic of cause and effect but any association—such as synchronicity.

In simpler words, in a shamanic journey like Dorothy's there are no accidents. It was her deep desire all along to overcome the power of her conditional shadow self, and her victory is a cause for celebration. This in fact happens when the members of the Wicked Witch's guard are released from bondage by Dorothy's deed. "All hail Dorothy!" becomes the cry, signifying further the integration of previously sleeping or repressed aspects of her identity.

Oz Uncovered

Once again it is Toto who saves the day when Dorothy and her friends are granted a second audience with the Wizard. Toto exposes Oz as the man behind the curtain, and the wizard must then confess that he, too, is a failure. A simple man from Kansas, he once blew into Oz on a hot air balloon from a state fair and was accepted as a

wizard by the inhabitants of the city. Nonetheless, he does have so-
lutions to the travelers' problems. He rightly determines that what
Scarecrow, Tin Man and Lion need is recognition for the qualities
they already have but deem missing, and accordingly awards them a
diploma, a heart-shaped medal and a testimonial. Dorothy's need is
also something she already possesses, namely the way home to her
true Self, and the Wizard offers to escort her back to Kansas himself
in his hot air balloon, stating that he had always intended to return
one day anyway.

Identifying the Wizard as a man from Kansas points the way to
seeing what role the Wizard plays in Dorothy's process of transformation. As a reflection from waking consciousness he is none other
than Professor Marvel, but in her dream state he actually has several
identities, each one of them significant.

Besides being the Wizard, the same actor, Frank Morgan, plays
the doorman, the cabbie and the palace guard in Oz. A doorman is
one who presides over the opening (or closing) of a doorway, which
in Dorothy's case refers to hitherto unrealized parts of her greater
identity. Likewise a cab driver provides and guides the vehicle for
traveling, which also leads to new places. Finally, as a protector of
the inner sanctum, the palace guard must be won over, and it is
highly significant (as we shall see) that this happens through the
emotional expression of tears. And finally Oz himself, as what has
been journeyed to with so much hope, provides the final key to
Dorothy's transformation.

That the Wizard is a man is interesting, but not only from the
psycho-sexual viewpoint that relates psychic wholeness to a conscious identification with all aspects of one's human experience, both
masculine and feminine. Maleness in our culture often signifies authority, and it is exactly this, the authority or empowerment of her
divine or true Self that Dorothy is after. Oz, in this regard, is only

another gateway, a further level of unfoldment to be reached before Dorothy can truly get where she is going. After all, despite her hopes, the Wizard can't really take her home, which is why this myth of transcendence is a far cry from patriarchally-dependent fairly tales like *Cinderella*.

In fact, there are no male heroes in the film. Dorothy is both the seeker and the sought after, and the path to her empowerment is naturally feminine. In this regard it is significant that all of the male characters in her dream state become at some stage quite emotional, and contrary to cultural norms these men cry quite readily— and like the palace guard even uncontrollably.

No Place Like Home

So once more, just when Dorothy thinks she has finally made it, another trial presents itself. And again it is Toto who inspires the complication. All set to sail off with the defrocked Wizard to Kansas, Dorothy is forced to choose between her ego self and her potential wholeness when Toto bounds out of the balloon after a cat. This is significant not only because Toto (as a representation of Dorothy's total being) repeatedly defies confinement, but also because it mirrors in a clever way the same choice she had to make back in Kansas: to remain bound to the limits of external authority or to strike out on her own to discover who she truly is—even when it is hugely inconvenient. But Dorothy, a mythic seeker, never hesitates about following her heart, leaving the incompetent Wizard (who can't even navigate his own hot air balloon) to be blown haphazardly back to Kansas.

Of course Kansas isn't really Dorothy's destination anyway. So as soon as she has gathered Toto back into her arms, who should appear but Glinda, the Good Witch of the North. Glinda has all along been the wise and loving reflection of Dorothy's true power and good-ness, and she has come to inform Dorothy that she has always had the power to return home. Dorothy, of course, had to learn this for herself in order to understand the responsibility and scope of her new empowerment, which she then expresses in the characteristi-cally encoded manner of the film. Above all, she asserts, she has come to understand that she doesn't have to look for her heart's desire anywhere but in her own back yard, and if it isn't there then she never really lost it in the first place.

This bit of what superficially seems to be trite Hollywood senti-mentality is profound for at least two reasons. On the one hand, it points to the realization that her happiness is to be found where she already is, that acceptance of the transcendent self in the moment is the key to inner peace and fulfillment. And if she ever does feel a lack or longing of any kind she now knows to look no further than her own backyard, which is an area behind (or unconscious to) the house which has become her identity. This reveals that Dorothy has intuitively grasped that the total self is reflected in a process of be-coming and cannot be contained by rigid forms or structures. In fact, when the ego self attempts to contain identity in restrictive forms, the essential or transcendent self will take every opportunity to es-cape confinement—just like Toto.

As for the second half of Dorothy's statement of what she's learned, that if there's anything her heart desires that can't be found in her own backyard it was something she never lost in the first place, the seeming illogic of her words clearly displays the essence of our de-sires. We seek what we already have within us, and it is when we don't recognize this that we are most lost. We are, in other words, potentially already happy and at peace. It is our perceptions of who we are that keep us from realizing and experiencing such content-ment. So when we believe that the recognition and empowerment we thirst for is unattainable—in other words if we somehow believe our value and identity are to be found outside of ourselves—then we will experience the despair created by our fearful perceptions of lack.

At Glinda's pronouncement that Dorothy is about to go home, if that is what she wants, Dorothy says her good-byes, and after tapping her ruby slippers together three times and repeating "There's no place like home," she finds herself back in her old bed in the black-and-white world of waking consciousness. But she is no longer the same Dorothy, though she may appear that way to her family and friends. She tries to explain to them about her journey to the kingdom of Oz, yet all they know and see is their familiar Dorothy so her tale is met with loving but condescending indulgence. Characteristically, she protests: "It wasn't a dream! It was a place. A real, truly live place! Doesn't anyone believe me?" But she quickly sees that they do not, and for the moment that really doesn't matter. She is back among her loved ones, and she takes the opportunity to tell them how much she loves them all. Then, with Toto back in her arms, Dorothy vows to never, ever leave home again.

Good Folks, Bad Wizards

The movie ends here, but in essence Dorothy's true path, and the healing of her core wound, has really only just begun. The others may not accept the literalness of her journey, but they will certainly begin to experience the transformed Dorothy as she demonstrates her newly found identification with her empowered, transcendent self. In fact it is certain that there will be more and perhaps even greater trials and crises in Dorothy's life now that she has come into her power, and it is equally clear that she will most likely face them bravely and with an unshakeable confidence in the validity of her process. After all, her journey was often fun, full of excitement and adventure, and no matter how gray her waking consciousness may appear she sees that Kansas is no longer Kansas any-more. With her return a new journey has begun for Dorothy, for all transcendent endings are simultaneously beginnings as that which has come before becomes part of what has been newly created.

Dorothy's next adventure will involve the emotional healing that creates the true Self in the world, and at this point we can only speculate how that story may go. We can, however, contrast her two worlds in order to uncover even more of the magic of transcendent process. To begin with, the characters of Oz, as mirrors or reflections of Dorothy, give a clear indication of what was needed for Dorothy's self-discovery. Yet when we place the two worlds alongside one an-other it becomes immediately clear that the principal characters do not all have correspondences. Neither Aunt Em nor Uncle Henry appear as anything other than their waking consciousness selves, and Glinda isn't at all anticipated in the opening scenes.

What this suggests in the case of Aunt Em and Uncle Henry is that these are still significant aspects of Dorothy that must be tran-scended, just as a child must always in some sense go beyond its parents in order to become a true individual. As for Glinda, this Good Witch of the North represents Dorothy's innate strength and goodness, as already mentioned. But Glinda is also more than that, for turning once again to Native American perspectives we see that Glinda represents Dorothy's starting point on the transcendent path. In the traditions of the Native American Plains Indians, a human soul is said to come into this life from one of the four directions, bringing with it the perceptions and strengths of that direction to help as the challenges of the other directions of the circle are en-countered on the spiritual walk of the Medicine Wheel.

As a model of the transcendent process or path this applies un-cannily well to Dorothy, who as a native of the Great Plains meets up with the Wicked Witches of the East and West as she undergoes a shamanic journey. Borrowing the terms used in Hyemeyohsts

Storm's *Seven Arrows* for the Medicine Wheel, it is possible to understand Dorothy's journey to Oz from this perspective of her ancestral land. For as Storm points out, each of us has not only a Beginning Place on the Medicine Wheel, but also a particular Medicine Animal, which in Dorothy's case is Toto, or the medicine of the dog as discussed earlier. These two things form the Beginning Gift from the Great Spirit.

So Dorothy, drawing on the initiative of Toto and the Great Power or medicine of the North, which is wisdom, gains insight into the medicines of illumination (East) and introspection (West) as she overcomes their negative forces in the guises of the Wicked Witches. The direction that remains of course is the south, and it is certain that headstrong Dorothy will one day need to learn the lessons of surrender to heartfelt innocence that this direction has to teach.

And of course Dorothy is not yet finished with the other directions; she has only begun her conscious walk. This can be seen even in the figure of Glinda, who though good and wise is also somewhat unbalanced and needs the strengths and warmth of the other directions to be fully grounded. Dorothy's potential self, in fact, is greater than the sum of these individual perceptions, for the wholeness she may experience as an emotionally mature or even emotionally enlightened adult will include and point beyond all the Great Powers of the Medicine Wheel.

Dorothy's status as an orphan again bears consideration for how it emphasizes how different she is from those around her. As a shaman, wizard or healer her role is partly one of an outsider, yet this too is a matter of perception and must be overcome in order for her to be fully empowered. Learning to live simultaneously in both worlds may instruct Dorothy in the ways of being a true wizard, but this will only happen if she is able to grow with an expanding sense of the wonder and blessings of life. For Dorothy is no different than any other human being; she has simply discovered the playfulness and wisdom of her transcendent self. And she must remember that just like the Wizard, her disbelieving family members are good folks, just bad wizards. This in fact is the underlying message of *The Wizard of Oz* when viewed for its lessons on the path of transcendence. We are all reflections of one another, and even in what may appear to be the darkest of times or the most difficult of walks the power to transcend and rise to the challenges of greater love lies within—and is present in each moment.

And of course what applies to the transcendent journey of an individual holds equally for the collective journey we are undergoing as a society and as communities. In this regard, *The Wizard of Oz* speaks to us in many ways. Most significantly, the film resonates in our hearts for being emblematic of the emergent feminine that is being consciously and unconsciously called forth as the antidote to the self-destructive harshness and heartlessness of our world as it stands. In our waking consciousness creations of reality we are critically out of balance with the loving intention of Life, and the degree to which we embrace the rise of the feminine will determine how rocky the road of healing will be.

The stark contrast between the black-and-white world of Kansas and the almost hallucinogenic technicolor of the Land of Oz is another of the essential ways this film speaks to us collectively. Not only is a playful, harmonious world more fun, it is also intrinsically beautiful. And it is beauty, as an aspect of the universal feminine (not gender specific), that is so sorely missing from our lives. Beauty, or more specifically *radiance*, is the quality of balanced, open-hearted living, and we would be wise to adopt higher standards of beauty both in our environments and in our relations with all beings. Beauty, in this sense, is not an aesthetic of form, but a cultivated quality of spirit. To walk in beauty, which is an expression of the native peoples of our land, is to be truly at home in the world—which is what every seeker's heart desires.

Chapter Three Main Points

1.   Each obstacle or challenge we face asks the same question: Who are You? Practical Application: Understanding that Life is challenging us to overcome our lies of unknowing and fears of unworthiness strengthens us and gives us more courage to act from the centerpoint of our being.

2.   The full flowering of love can only happen in our lives once we've claimed and experienced our own divinity. Practical Application: It is solely our own responsibility to claim ourselves, and we must learn that judgment against Life is misplaced and self-defeating.

3.   Our true creative potential can only be unlocked by unconditional self-approval. Practical Application: Recognizing how much we hold ourselves back from our creative nature through self-limiting ideas and self-negating behaviors empowers us to change and grow.

4.   The adventure of becoming is a process of self-discovery, emotional healing, and creative expression. Practical Application: Having a map of the process for realizing our potentials clarifies our personal path.

5.   Stories, whether personal or communal, are always about personal experiences of growth and transformation. Practical Application: Seeing our own life history as a story full of symbols and dynamic forces leading us toward greater meaning and transcendence allows us to take a step back and pay closer attention to how Life is guiding us.

6.   Making sense of our dreams means learning to apply associative reasoning to the emotional content of a dream. Practical Application: As bridges between the conscious and unconscious,

dreams offer a golden opportunity to recognize emotional tensions that are in need of resolution.

7. *The Wizard of Oz* is a cultural myth, acting as a collective dream to instruct us in the ways of personal growth and transcendence. Practical Application: Understanding how story functions for us communally brings greater appreciation for how important such stories are, as well as for how less affirming stories can lead to spiritual and creative frustration.

8. Transcendent growth is dependent upon how fully we actualize our inner identity in the outside world. Practical Application: Knowing of our potential is only the first step—from there we must bring it into form if we desire to find our greatest happiness.

9. The conditional world of blame exists solely in our own wounded hearts. Practical Application: Realizing that faulting others for our feelings or perceived failures is a sign that we are temporarily trapped in our conditional woundedness can motivate us to seek out the source of our self-judgment.

10. It is beauty, as an aspect of the universal feminine, that is sorely missing from our lives. Practical Application: We are wise to adopt higher standards of beauty for our environments and our relations with others.

Exercise for Experiential Understanding

This exercise will reveal how the powerful symbolism that underlies our family stories points us toward greater meaning, transcendence and connection in our lives. You will need pen and paper, and possibly a tape recorder.

The power of myth that we see in *The Wizard of Oz* is also active in our lives. Bringing this power forward and making it actively present involves looking a little more closely at the stories we tell to each other and ourselves. The first step is to identify a story that has mythic potential—some story that defines a great change in life for the main character of the story, whether it's you or someone else. You may even wish to use a story that one of your parents or grandparents likes to tell. Good examples are: immigration stories, job or career change stories, birth stories, first meeting stories, and even stories about the death of someone close.

Next, either tape record or write out the story, making sure to put as many details as possible into this first telling. If you are using someone else's story, it's best to tape record because that gives you more freedom to ask questions for eliciting greater explanation and detail. Once you have a first version that more or less works, go through the story to identify both the key turning points in the story as well as anything that may work well as a symbol. Possible symbols include someone's dress (remember Dorothy's shoes), weather events, artifacts or keepsakes, coincidental happenings and even specific food items.

Before you go any further, identify the transcendent meaning of the story. What kind of change occurred in the main character, and why? How did s/he grow? Once you have established this meaning or lesson you must rework the story somewhat to bring that meaning forward, embellishing and adding significant details (events, new characters, props) where appropriate. Keep the flavor of the original story as much as possible, but also feel free to exercise your poetic license to change things around for greater effect. Try especially hard to emphasize and build up the turning points.

As soon as you feel ready, try your story out on family members or friends. Expect strong reactions from those also involved in the story, and use their feedback for further fine tuning. Remember, it's not really your story but a mythologized version of your story, so don't hold on too tightly to things that may need to be changed for greater effect. You'll also find that the more you tell the story, it will take on its own life as new details are magically added in the telling, or old details and story elements fall by the wayside.

You may even wish to rewrite several stories that are told and retold at family gatherings or among friends. The more you bring out the hidden mythic nature of these real life stories the more you will be asked to tell them, so be prepared for the spotlight!

Questions for Contemplation

On your journey to wholeness, your walk around the medicine wheel, what important qualities do you feel you are lacking or deficient in? Take enough time to honestly answer this question. Where do you feel you are not enough? To help you in this, think of any regrets you may have about your past, and try and determine what quality or qualities would have helped you in that time. Now for the hard part. Recognize that the quality or qualities you have identified are indeed already a part of you—or you wouldn't be able to recognize them. Who on your walk is a guide, a reflection for you of this quality? How will you create the conditions for these qualities to be revealed more fully in you?

Notes:

Emotional Healing

The unspoken truth of myths like *The Wizard of Oz* is that our black-and-white everyday world is one veil of perception away from a vibrantly colorful wonderland. Mystery and magic are the underpinnings of our existence, and if that is not our experience, the reason lies in the perceptive lens through which we view and create our lives. And until we can recognize that it is our own distorted sense of who we are that keeps us from living each moment for the gift it is, we will search in vain for something outside of ourselves to set us free.

In our sometimes frenzied quest for happiness we routinely overlook one crucial truth: we are already in touch with our happiness. Wonder, happiness, magic, love and mystery are who we are and have always been. This is true because at our being's very core we are nothing less than the very force of play and creation that has spawned universes and designed the intricate beauties of our world. That we do not know to revel in our creative genius is part of the play, a creative constraint that first forms our potentials before it asks to be transcended—much like the butterfly that must force itself out of the cocoon to find liberation and display its radiant color.

Self-discovery is the first dawning of the realization that, like Dorothy, we are already home. We have seen—if only briefly—through the veil of our misperception and gratefully discovered that we have within us the source of our magical creation. In a very real sense, such understanding empowers us to be more consciously involved in the creation of our lives. Moreover, with this realization comes the insight that in a very real way we are the source of our own suffering, and from there we can begin to truly heal.

Such self-discovery also wakes us up to the fact that we live in a self-reflective universe. Our internal truth is always being reflected back to us, but it is only when we connect to the source of our creation that we can begin to understand that all of Life is not only reflecting our beauty but also working to create the conditions necessary for our greatest possible display of that beauty. Life wants nothing more than for us to delight in our being.

Sometimes it feels nearly impossible to accept the truth that in this larger sense, whatever is in our life is there to inspire or even force the growth of our self-acceptance, which is the necessary foundation for our creative expression and realization of greater love. It seems easier to believe that Life is conspiring against us to make our lives as difficult as possible, throwing every possible obstacle into our paths. What makes us doubt the cooperative efforts of Life is our core wounding, for it influences us to unconsciously (or even consciously) believe that we are not worthy of what we desire. The truth is that we are not only absolutely worthy of lives of magic and wonder, but also that our desires themselves are to some degree products of our wounding, limiting us to desires and dreams that are far below our true potential.

Because what we feel we want and deserve is significantly influenced by our core wounding, if we indeed wish to find our greatest happiness we must learn one of Life's most difficult lessons. We must give up control. We must accept the fact that our wounding is tripping us up, making us take steps backward for all steps we take forward. This of course does not mean that we must give up action or give our power away to something or someone else. Rather, we must learn to work in concert with Life, and to accept that when it comes right down to it, Life will offer us exactly what we need at all times to shape and guide us to our greatest potentials, for our greatest displays of love and creativity are also Life's fullest expressions of human joy.

The idea of giving up control quite naturally causes some misgivings, so it is useful to know that what we must do is give up our need for absolute control. (This can also be experienced as the need to be right.) The simple explanation for this is that in order for the simple or false ego to evolve into the transcendent ego, we must accept that mystery, or the unknowable, is at the core of our identity. Doing this allows us to make the crucial connection between mystery within and mystery outside—they are the same divine mystery. From there, the ego can begin to accept its higher role as the facilitator of heartfelt transcendence.

We have all witnessed what happens when this development from simple ego to transcendent ego gets stalled, or completely derailed. The false ego becomes greedy for control, desperate in its attempts to find some satisfaction. Yet without that conscious, direct link to the mystery within and the mystery outside—and the resultant glimpse of one's own divinity, there will be no satisfaction possible. The insatiable thirst for satisfaction becomes the source of one or more control trips: predatory sexuality, greed for fame or fortune, or domination games of endless variety. And it is important to know that even once self-discovery has happened, and we surrender to the mysteries within and all around us as being a central part of who we are, without completing our emotional healing we will also be caught up in some kind of futile search for satisfaction and control.

Creating the Authentic Self

For the most part, it is customary for us to regard any aspect of ourselves that we do not like, whether we call it our shadow, our dark side, our karma, our weakness, our sin, or our wounding, as what we would like to get rid of—preferably as soon as possible. If only we were free of our anger or our loneliness, we believe, we would then be able to live up to our expectations for ourselves and have more meaningful, rewarding lives. If only we could be stronger, we think, then we could stop doing whatever it is that hurts us or others and finally find some peace.

There are two main problems with this common approach. First of all, such an attitude sees the wounding as something external, or at least something that can be surgically removed. The reality is that our wounding is woven into the very fabric of our sense of identity. An equally serious problem with this sort of attitude is that it causes us to resist or deny the experiences of our wounding. This means that we either look to others or to Life as the source of our pain, or that we deny the pain altogether, thereby creating armoring that desensitizes or even deadens us. And the consequences of seeing our wounding as negative (or even evil), feed right into a kind of crisis management that has us turning around and around to put out the fires that won't stop springing up wherever we turn—without our ever being able to determine their source.

The fundamental flaw in seeing our wounding as negative is that such a perspective contradicts the fact that Life is presenting us at all times with exactly what is needed and necessary for the highest creative expressions of our being. Our wounding, therefore, is not something to be avoided or removed, but is designed to function as what will inspire our evolution and healing. Beyond our basic need to physically survive, it is our wish to be happy and creatively fulfilled that drives us, and the dynamic of our emotional wounding provides the inner tension that leads us toward what we know to be our highest truth. In short, our wounding is not what defines our identity but is what we can use to consciously fuel our transcendence. In a sense, our wounding is a measure of our potentials for love and creative expression.

Seen in this way, healing is nothing less than the way in which we create the authentic self. As our wounding is eased, the energetic tension of the core wound dynamic becomes directly translated into the creation of a sense of self that is in alignment with the truth of our absolute worthiness and divinity. The result is that the new world we begin to create for ourselves is increasingly a reflection of our innate goodness since we are no longer denying or negating who we are. And the most tangible change we experience from the easing of our wound is that our lives begin to feel more joyous than burdensome. And the common misperception that no matter what we do there will always be an equal balance of suffering and joy in our lives comes from the experience of the simple or false ego, not the transcendent ego.

Another way to understand this process is to say that the self-limiting and self-negating drives of the ego are through our emotional healing gradually reduced, leading us to greater identification with the transcendent ego. And the transcendent ego, unlike the false ego created in the early stages of our emotional evolution, allows for the divine nature of our being to be consciously and graciously integrated into our sense of self. This surrender of control is precisely what we need to make the personal connection between Life's efforts to inspire us to our potential and the continuously emergent self that is created from within. In simpler words, our true, or transcendent, ego embraces the essential mystery of our becoming, which means that our self-limiting concepts of self are overcome.

For example, let us imagine a young man who struggles with anger. This anger is rooted in deep frustration, and he is unable to stop himself both from lashing out at others and from the feelings of shame that follow such outbursts. His anger is the outward expression of his wounding, his sense of unworthiness and lack, which he doesn't know to heal. In his mind he feels that he has a right to be angry because of all that has happened to him, especially the way he was treated by his father. Such anger, he feels, is just the way he is because of his history, and there is nothing to be done but try and control it. His ego or conditional self, in other words, creates an identity for him that explains his anger as an unchangeable and barely manageable aspect of his character.

From the view of the transcendent self there is a very different story going on. The young man's anger is fierce because of how tightly the self has been defined, leaving no room for the possibility that this anger is a creative force unable to find its positive creative expression. The feelings of shame and regret are the key to emotional healing and creation of the authentic self because they are where his underlying self-negation can be touched. Rather than controlling the anger, which rationalizes it as a given force to be dealt with, the source of the anger as the young man's self-loathing must be consciously experienced by him so that it may be healed. Once there is some experience of relief through transcendence, the young man can begin to learn how Life will cooperate with him to create his authentic self.

The need for the surrender of control that marks the difference between our false, self-limiting self and our authentic, transcendent self cannot be overstated. In the woundedness of our false self we mistakenly feel that we know who we are and what we need. We can even seem to find proof of these things in our worldly successes and in our accomplishments, which reinforce, often self-righteously, the sense that we know what is best for us and our happiness. The reality is that we are blinded by the web of deceit created by our deepest sense of unworthiness. That we do not necessarily feel unworthy in the identity we have created by the false ego doesn't matter. The real proof of our core wounding is in our struggling and in our suffering.

Confident, seemingly self-satisfied and accomplished people are shocked when they discover the truth of their core wounding. Usually this happens through some kind of personal crisis, although occasionally it can happen through an experience of insight. Often, the so-called mid-life crisis is brought about by the false self's inability to bring about the happiness it promised. The job, the family, the activities are all in place, but there is still a deep sense of unease, of despair. In a desperate attempt to make up for what feels like a loss of time, values become reshuffled and an effort is made to create a new life. Unless this new life is grounded in the truth of the transcendent self or ego, it will simply be one false self built on top of an earlier false self.

True self-discovery means realizing that on the most fundamental level of your identity you have been had. What you thought to be true about yourself and the world are simply wrong, and there's no way to avoid the truth that it is your own wounding or sense of self that has caused your suffering. That is the reality of genuine self-discovery. Even further, such self-discovery enlightens you to the fact that this is everyone's story. We are all playing out the same journey of self-creation that begins in delusion about the truth of the self. And the only true path forward after genuine self-discovery is the way of emotional healing, where the lies of the false ego are transformed into a truly new identity, the authentic self.

Dynamics of Emotional Healing

The first thing to understand about the self-delusion of the ego or false self is that it is completely natural, and is the consequence of our core wounding working through the metaphoric nature of our sense-making. As discussed in the second chapter, the core wound tension between our divine knowingness and the reflected conditionality of our humanity leads us to favor conditionality in the formation of our sense of self, or ego. This is exactly as it should be, for this set-up puts into place the creative constraints that will be transcended when following our self-discovery we begin to express our true natures. Again much like the butterfly, who must struggle out of the cocoon in order to set its wings in place, the tension of our core wounding provides us with the energy and direction for the creation of our authentic self.

The pacing of our journeys toward self-discovery is largely determined by the metaphoric or associative way that our consciousness works. To start with, seeing ourselves, and therefore our wounding, is difficult because in a very real sense we are what we are trying to see. When we add to this the understanding that our sense-making relies on making connections or associations with what is already known, the result is that our tendency will always be toward retaining what we already believe to be the truth about ourselves. This is one reason why people generally hear only what they want to hear, and generally seem to find confirmation for what they already feel to be true—even in new situations and surroundings.

This emphasizes why it is so useful to understand not only how we make sense of things, but also how the three modes of our experience (body, emotion and mind) function and interact. The functional relationship between emotion and mind, for example, is especially important to understand for how we see and understand ourselves. This is because the stories we have about who we are and what Life is all about will always contain within them our core wounding. Our wounding, in other words, can be difficult if not seemingly impossible to see because of how involved it is in the identity and Life purpose stories that make sense to us.

If, for example, because of our core wounding we unconsciously accept as true the self-negating lies of our conditional self or false ego that envision us as unworthy, the world and our personal identity will only seem to make sense in ways that assume that our struggles and suffering are simply a fact of Life. This "real life" version of Life is correct to acknowledge that suffering is a natural and unavoidable aspect of human experience, but it is our deeply held resentment, anger and self-diminishment that makes this version of reality feel emotionally right—and blinds us to the incompleteness and despair of our outlook.

Whatever story we have to explain who we are and what Life is all about, our emotional wounding will be woven into its very fabric, giving us a false sense of the story's rightness because of how it reflects back to us what we unconsciously deem to be correct. If at the foundation of our emotional being we accept as true our insignificance or our ugliness, only those stories that in some way make sense of that emotional belief will feel right to us. That means only those views of the world that support such beliefs will be seriously entertained, which only serves to further solidify those beliefs because they appear to be objectively evident in the world outside.

The self-fulfilling nature of our core beliefs, especially about ourselves and our worthiness, has been well documented. Yet it is less understood how these beliefs are constructions of mind *and* emotion. Mind, in fact, imaginatively constructs its stories based on the emotional terrain, as just explained. But since transcendence is a matter of emotion, not mind, challenging self-limiting core beliefs is best approached by simultaneously relaxing our attachment to our stories (no matter how sacred they may seem) and focusing on the emotions that support or contain the belief.

Fortunately, the very design of our being points a way toward loosening the grip that mind can have over our emotional development as well as over our emotional experience. Each of our experiential modes is not separate, but must rather be understood as a different focus or face of the same holistic being. This means that all of our modes are interconnected and interdependent. Yes, we may have personal tendencies or preferences for one or another of our modes, but they all reflect and in one sense contain the others. And since we know that mind can hide our emotional wounding and also restrict our emotional experience, we can facilitate change by developing and working with the other two modes of our experience. As healing occurs, mind, body and emotion will naturally find greater balance if all three modes were involved in the healing.

Finding and maintaining balance between body, emotion and mind is foundational to our well being. Life is swirling with energy and change, and so are we. Imbalance comes about when for whatever reason we ignore or resist some facet of our experience. And for the most part, in our society we primarily resist our emotional experience, and retreat either into the physical or into mind. What results, of course, is disease and unhappiness.

Our greatest reason for resisting the depths of our emotional experience is that we are under the hypnotic spell of our false self. We falsely believe that our negative feelings are caused by others or are the result of Life's unfairness or inherent difficulty. (Remember, the false self believes that it is in control and can do no or little wrong.) We choose to see our negative or unpleasant feelings as being unjustly caused by someone or something—or even by our inadequate selves. We then hold on to this mind-story as an unassailable truth, and in doing so we effectively limit our growth and throw ourselves out of balance. Or, we mistakenly believe that someone or something can make us happy. This effectively blinds us to how we have enslaved ourselves and our happiness to something outside of our-selves—which is a certain recipe for crisis and suffering.

Our habits of resisting and misunderstanding our emotional ex-perience are reflected strongly in our other two modes of experience, the body and the mind. Our emotional wounds are clearly held in the body (once we know how and where to look), and they are also clearly evident in the stories our minds use to explain away or justify our negative emotions. And all of this occurs simply because we do not understand how our negative emotional experiences are the energy, the growing edge, of our becoming and should be positively integrated into our overall experience.

Emotional Integration

When we understand and accept that emotion is the realm of our personal truth, we immediately face a crucial question: What should we do with our negative emotions?

No one wants to feel pain, and the pain of emotional distress can be as debilitating as any physical injury. In fact emotional distress can lead to physical pain and so-called mystery illnesses. But when we understand that our emotional distress can always be traced back to our core wounding, it becomes clear that how we react to our emotional suffering is vitally important. In the overall design of Life, we are intended to heal our core wounding so that we can truly know and express the love for life and living that is the source of our being. For this reason, we must learn to accept the fact that even in our most extreme emotional turmoil there exists a means for grace-ful healing.

This can be a difficult truth. Our emotional pain seems at times to cry out for drama—and we often are quick to oblige. At other times it may all seem like too much, and we reach for the handiest sedative—whether it's television, alcohol, sleep, food or drugs. And of course there are also those moments when we are most inclined to silently suffer, to tear ourselves down for what we have done—or for our absolute stupidity. These responses, representative of the three defensive reaction patterns that we reach for out of habit, will of course never really satisfy us, for they don't reach to the root cause of our distress.

These three defensive reaction patterns—attack, desensitize (camouflage) and withdraw—are familiar to all of us. We use them all, alone or in combination, virtually each time we are emotionally hurt in some way. Not surprisingly, these are also recognizable in nature as the hard-wired responses to danger of fight or flight and camouflage/play dead. Because of our higher level of consciousness, however, we do not have to accept these ingrained responses. We are in fact evolutionarily expected to transcend them. And the best way to begin to transcend these patterns is wonderfully simple: mindful sensory experience.

Balance is the key. We are designed to evolve, so really all we have to do is bring all of ourselves to our experience in order to fully activate our transcendent natures. This means integrated experience, or in emotional terms, emotional integration. Mindful sensory experience therefore is exactly what is called for when we are emotionally distressed. The mindfulness part simply means to watch, to witness our experience so that we can recognize the patterning and programming as well as to allow space for the emotional energy to flow. (Witnessing signals that we are greater than the distress, not identified with it.) The sensory experience part means that while we are mindfully witnessing our distress we make sure that we experience it as fully in our bodies as we can.

This evolved response to our emotional distress, mindful sensory experience, needs further explanation. First of all, we must understand that transcendence is our nature. What this means is that the question of what we are to do with our suffering is somewhat misleading. Yes, we can pay attention and make sure we are physically feeling our emotions—and this is the wisest approach. However, the real doing that is going on, whether or not we are consciously assisting, is beyond our control and belongs to the inherent mystery of our becoming and the wonder of Life. In truth, we cannot heal ourselves; we can only be healed. It is the same as when we plant a seed. We do not actually grow the plant; we simply provide the best conditions for it to realize its transcendent potential—to go from seed to full-grown plant.

This means that when we are in emotional distress, the best way to regain balance and consciously assist in the energy of our becoming that is currently in the form of emotional pain is to provide the best possible conditions for transcendent growth. Transcendence, as stated before, involves going beyond yet also including what is or has come before. Mindful sensory experience does this by doing two things simultaneously. First of all, it brings the fullness of our being to our experience by consciously including the other modes of our experience, mind and body, to our emotional distress. Secondly, mindful sensory experience assists, rather than resists, the forces of our becoming.

Our standard responses to emotional pain, the three defensive reaction patterns mentioned earlier, are coping habits that in effect resist our emotional evolution and growth—much like driving with our foot on the brake. Taking our foot off the brake not only makes driving easier, it also saves a lot of wear and tear on our energy system. In addition, assisting with the forces of our emotional evolution means that we will make some headway in healing our core wounding.

Once we stop resisting, we will begin to recognize the ways we are defending and protecting ourselves—when in reality our unconditional worthiness makes such defensiveness unnecessary. The truth is, we are absolutely as worthy as all others, and when we feel of-fended—or any kind of lack of acceptance or approval—the source is not outside of ourselves but in the ways and beliefs of our condi-tional or false ego.

Of course embracing rather than resisting the forces of our be-coming still involves action. We still must make choices that will provide optimal conditions for our continued growth, but these choices will be conscious ones and not the habitual responses of our unconscious defensive reactions. And mindful sensory experience also takes practice. There will be times when we will react uncon-sciously with full force and won't have the time or presence of mind to recognize the dynamics of our own wounding. With practice, how-ever, we will recognize and experience the results of mindful sensory experience, and this will sharpen our awareness and inspire us to embrace our transcendent becoming even more. To assist with this, the exercises following each chapter will be useful for building the skills to make mindful sensory experience easier to implement at all times.

Body, Mind and Balance

Using mindful sensory experience to find and maintain the bal-ance necessary for graceful transcendent evolution gives us an approach to our emotional distress and suffering that will begin to heal our core wounding. This approach also has far-reaching impli-cations that need to be further explored if we wish to take full advantage of how we can more consciously assist in our personal growth and emotional evolution.

The first place we can discover the power of mindful sensory ex-perience is in the body. In one sense, our body mode of experience is the most primary way we have of experiencing Life and who we are.

Our bodies must be properly cared for simply for us to survive, and if we wish to realize our potentials for love and creativity we must learn to find balance and harmony between body, mind and emotion. In terms of emotional healing, what this means is that we must learn to recognize the emotional component of all our physical pain and dis-ease.

The mind/body connection has been widely documented (the growing field is called psychoneuroimmunology) and popularized to the point where we are all aware and accepting of how thoughts and attitude not only affect our healing when we are sick, but also affect our immune system and therefore how susceptible we are to sickness in the first place. What is generally less understood, however, is how our bodies speak to us in emotional terms. Because of the holistic nature of our being, distress in the body will reflect emotional distress, and vice versa. Of course our minds are also part of the system, which means that our ideas about who we are and what Life is all about will also be reflected in the body, but since it is our emotional experience that most directly reveals our core emotional wounding it is generally more efficient to work with emotional distress as it is reflected either in the body or in the mind. (Moreover, emotional energy, as the middle energy in terms of density, has more immediate physical effects than mind energy does and can therefore more quickly ease physical discomfort.)

What this means in practical terms is that we can view any physical ailment as being reflective to some degree of our emotional wounding. Whether it's a cold we have or even a sprain, this experience will also be emotional, and we can practice mindful sensory experience as a way to integrate any negative emotional energy associated with our physical ailment. Doing this will in fact accelerate physical healing as well as emotional healing.

Emotional wounding or emotional issues are sometimes viewed as being the cause of all physical suffering, and specific correlations have been mapped out between diseases or body areas and psycho-emotional issues. While such mapping can be helpful for eliciting responses and gaining some clarity between mind/body connections, it should also be understood that each of us is unique, and our specific correlations between emotional issues and physical ailments will be equally unique.

The body, however, does speak to us metaphorically—and sometimes with amazing clarity. This is shown sometimes even in our language, which equates physical postures with emotional ways of being. A stiff upper lip refers to an emotional attitude, as do hunched shoulders, a head held high and a spring in one's step. Butterflies in the stomach and clenched jaws also reflect emotional experiences and attitudes—to the point that chronic negative emotional experiences will begin to mold our musculature to the holding or resistance pattern. For such postural manifestation of emotional issues it is possible to unwind the emotional holding that keeps the posture locked, leading to greater physical as well as emotional freedom.

In addition to working with physical experience to access and heal emotional wounding, gaining greater insight into the dynamics of emotional wounding is a way to further maximize the effectiveness of the mindful sensory experience approach to healing and emotional evolution. It is useful to understand, for example, how the core emotional needs of safety, nurturance and guidance are a part of our emotional evolution journey and therefore a part of our wounding.

Safety

Our most basic need, both physically and emotionally, is for safety (correlative to the body mode of experience). Without protection from the elements and from the dangers of the world that can threaten our survival, as children we would have no hope for making it even to our first birthday. As we grow in the ability to care for ourselves this need for safety will become less physically urgent, but our emotional need to be safe will remain with us throughout our lives. Indeed feeling safe is a prerequisite for the true opening of our hearts, and without that we will never experience our true nature.

Understandably, emotional wounding that results from safety issues will be deep within our being and may take time and patience to heal. The human heart, however, is capable of complete transcendence, and this means that even deep emotional wounding around basic safety and emotional security issues can be healed. What's needed is a correct identification of the wounding, and a graceful approach that uses a balanced and integrated method of body, mind and emotion. As in all cases of healing, once steps are taken, Life will respond with the appropriate help.

Emotional patterns and experiences involving safety issues are often due to physical abuse or actual physical abandonment. Depending on the temperament of the child, poverty and frequent relocation may also engender safety and emotional security issues, as may divorce or the death of a family member. In all of these cases and others, there will be chronic feelings of insecurity that don't seem to lessen even in the face of material security or even abundance. It is possible, in fact, that the individual may become overly concerned with material security, and may have the sense of never having enough physical comfort. With more serious safety wounding, chronic fears of disaster may also be present, as well as agoraphobia and other fears of the outside world or other people.

Ultimately, the only true safety and emotional security comes from the experience of Life's ability and intention to provide all that is needed for our self-discovery and loving creative expression. This means that the healing of safety issues should include very clear and intentional ways for developing one's experience of being supported by Life, including the discovery and development of one's passion-ate life purpose.

Nurturance

The second core need that we all have, both physically and emo-tionally, is for nurturance, which is corelative to the emotion mode of experience. Not only do we require food to sustain us physically, we also need love and kindness expressed to us through touch and with words and behavior. Without such nurturance we will never thrive, let alone survive.

The emotional wounding that occurs when we are not adequately nurtured is profound, for it contributes to and intensifies the forma-tion of our false self, the unconscious part of us who believes that we are not worthy of such nurturance. When our early experiences are of fear or withdrawal rather than loving nurturance, we may always feel like we can never get enough approval or praise. Or we may build a thick wall around our hearts so that no one can really touch us where we most need to be touched.

Deficiencies in emotional nurturance are common. Our parents were themselves deeply wounded, which increases the likelihood that it was challenging for them to give us the nurturance that we required. Emotional nurturance issues that we carry with us or de-velop in adulthood include fear of intimacy, acute defensiveness, dishonesty, and a variety of subtle manipulation habits we develop to try and get our emotional needs met. One key characteristic of emotional maturity is that we become aware of the source of such behaviors and make adequate choices to ensure that our needs are met in an unconditional and ecological (win/win) way.

Guidance

The third of our basic or core emotional needs is for guidance, correlative to the mind/imagination mode of experience. In emotional terms, guidance is what makes us aware of who we are and leads us to greater expression of that identity. Learning manners and social rules are of course types of guidance as well, but what we are most looking for is for someone to recognize us for who we truly are, to guide us to our talents and therefore our passion for life. To some degree we will of course get some true idea of who we are from our parents and from our families, and yet we are also often thrown a lot of interference in the forms of expectations and beliefs that have little if anything to do with our deepest truths.

Naturally, guidance and misguidance comes from our society as well as our families. We are constantly bombarded with images and messages that tell us that we are not good enough as we are, that we need to be this or that or have this or that in order to be worthy of being accepted. Very rarely, in relative terms, do we have experiences where we are truly seen as being fully worthy, as is, in the moment. And yet without this kind of recognition from others, it is much more difficult to find and maintain our true sense of identity. Without being seen for who we are and being guided to greater and greater expressions of that truth, we run the risk of never even knowing the beauty of our own being.

Unfortunately, this is more the norm than the exception. We are generally convinced of our inadequacy, and this makes it difficult not only to break free of our self-limiting sense-making, but also to serve as guides for others on their journeys. Having never received the guidance we needed to make wise choices for discovering and expressing our authentic selves, we become part of the distorted mirror that makes it difficult for others to discover and express their true being. This self-perpetuating reality of the blind leading the blind is a fair characterization of our present society.

Emotional issues resulting from inadequate guidance are probably too numerous to be succinctly listed, but may include addiction, rage, domestic violence, depression, low self-esteem and chronic frustration. In this arena our entire society is unfortunately severely deficient, as can be seen by how thoughtlessly we treat one another and our world. The reality is, we can only compassionately relate to others and to our surroundings to the degree that we know and experience our own self-worth, and for this we usually need to first be truly seen by another or by others and guided toward our highest potentials.

Self-Healing Through Positive Emotion

As made even clearer through identifying our basic or core emotional needs, we are all quite wounded to one degree or another. That this wounding is a natural part of our ego development and therefore a natural stage of our emotional evolution offers some comfort, however, for it also suggests that the healing of this wounding is also a potential part of our journey. In fact such healing, both individually and collectively, is our emotional destiny.

Ultimately, all emotional healing is self-healing. The emotional wounding that makes up the false self must be revealed for how it supports the lies of our unworthiness, and then we must create the authentic self to replace that false self from the inside out. Of course we can have help—and it is best to have help—in uncovering the deceptive and self-limiting ways of our false self, but we as individuals must do the work to release that wounding and express ourselves authentically.

The mindful sensory experience approach is extremely useful for revealing the wiles of the false self for purposes of healing, but we are wise to take on our healing from as many angles as possible in order to make thorough and quick work of it. And one often overlooked and underappreciated approach to emotional healing is through the discerning use of positive emotion. In other words, just as we can become mindfully aware of our negative emotions, we can also become mindfully aware of our positive emotions—and we can even devise strategies and practices for using positive emotion to facilitate growth and healing.

The use of positive affirmations is one method for applying positive emotions and positive attitudes to reprogram our subconscious and take some power away from the false self and its fear-based identity agenda. However, we must be careful when using such positive affirmations, for our purpose is to heal our core wounding, not simply cover it over with a layer of positive intention. Healing core wounding means tracing our fear-based or negative emotions to their root, and then witnessing their transformation into an empowered aspect of our authentic being. For this we'll need tools similar to positive affirmations, but with the added ability to go the distance in a mindful sensory experience way.

The Universal Love Meditation

It makes sense that for our emotional healing we should desire to tap into Life's most potent force: universal (unconditional) love. (We will use the term universal instead of unconditional because of its expansiveness, though universal and unconditional are interchangeable terms.) Nothing can lift us higher or inspire us more fully than the feelings and experience of absolute love. Such love is of course our highest good, the true north of all emotion. And since we are living expressions of Life, it is also already an intrinsic part of who we are. We don't really have to go anywhere to find love, for love is the hidden truth of all moments, ready to be revealed. This is the unbelievable secret of all mystery schools and all mystical and religious teachings. Love is there or here all the time; what fails us is our means for understanding and accessing this truth.

Part of the difficulty we have with feeling universal love in our lives at all times is that from the perspective of our sense-making, unconditional or universal love is a composite force, made up of many different strands or weaves. For this reason, it is useful for us to identify some of the main energies or weaves of absolute love so that we can recognize and activate them in our lives. The Universal Love Meditation is a method for doing exactly that—identifying five aspects of universal love, and then letting their energies heal our wounding through mindful sensory experience.

The five steps of the Universal Love Meditation are arranged in an order designed to maximize how the energies and feelings of love will combine and work together for graceful and profound healing and inspiration. What follows is a description of the five emotional elements of the meditation (or exercise, if you prefer), and at the end of the chapter there is a full explanation of the technique for self-healing, including hand positions and breathing. The first element is:

Gratitude

At the foundation of our experience of universal love is Gratitude. Gratitude is appreciation and profound thankfulness for all that supports us to live and love. Gratitude is a conscious, inward flowing acceptance of the gifts of Life, and our appreciation is a tacit recognition of our worthiness. Resistance to Gratitude comes in the many forms of resentment, which are indications and reflections of the hold our false self has on our being. Gratitude makes us aware of how Life works to shape and guide us to our greatest potentials for love and joyous creation.

Worthiness

The second element is Worthiness. What Worthiness teaches us is that in each moment we are saved, unconditionally redeemed and worthy. We have nothing to prove, and there is nothing to protect or defend against. Resistance to the truth of our unconditional worthiness at all times is the source of our striving and suffering. In each and every moment we are offered the choice of love, and how consciously aware of that choice we are is a measure of how deeply entrenched we are in the fears of the false self. Becoming aware of our divine Worthiness throughout our daily lives strengthens the hold of our authentic self so that we may eventually throw off the shackles of the conditional ego.

Praise

Following closely and building upon Gratitude and Worthiness comes the third element, Praise. Praise is the outward flowing acknowledgment and honoring for all of Life. It is the essence of creative energy and the natural outgrowth of joy. Upon finding the inherent happiness of our being, we are moved to express our wonder and even our awe at the unbounded source of love that emanates from all aspects and expressions of Life. Praise, as generosity of spirit, is itself a giving of that same love, and it is this realization that consciously connects our hearts to their source.

Compassion

The fourth element of the ladder is Compassion, a primary emotion of transcendence. In compassion we find our sympathy for all beings as we recognize our own suffering in others. Compassion is therefore not a diminishment of our own being in any way because our compassion is grounded in the realization of our worthiness. Though we may give to others out of compassion, such giving comes from our abundance, not from lack. Compassion is a primary emotion of transcendence because we understand that judgment is done out of ignorance; the truth is that just as we have made all choices in our lives based on our capabilities and knowledge, so it is for others as well. Regret and blame are two sides of the same lie of inadequacy and lack.

Trust

The final element of the Universal Love Meditation is perhaps also the most challenging: Trust. Trust is the understanding that each moment supports us and guides us to our highest realization and expression of our absolute worthiness and divinity. As we step forward in our authenticity, guided by our gratitude, sense of worthiness, praise and compassion, trust confirms that we will be met with what we need. Even in what may appear to be the most dire circumstances, the incessant questioning of Life about our true identity offers us the chance to experience the grace of our being. Trust is the key to our healing, and to the path of our highest good.

The Universal Love Meditation offers a multifaceted approach for healing through positive emotion. The Exercise for Experiential Understanding following this chapter will guide you through the five elements in a meditation exercise that can be done daily or as needed. Positive affirmations, guided imagery visualizations and focused meditations can also be extremely effective for healing through positive emotion when applied with the understandings of core wound dynamics.

Self as Other: The Mirror of Relationship

In terms of emotional healing, there is no area for greater potential growth than interpersonal relationship. Combined with our interdependence with one another, the core emotional wounding that is a natural development of our conditional ego sets the stage for all the emotional drama that anyone could want. This means that opportunities for healing are also relatively unlimited. To take advantage of these opportunities, we not only have to understand the dynamics of core wounding and healing that have already been presented, we also need to have a solid grasp of relationship mirroring, including triggering, projection and familial modeling.

The fact that our interpersonal relationships reflect ourselves back to us is a function of the overall self-reflection of consciousness. Our very sense of self depends on our sense of otherness. This basic interconnectedness of self and other at the root of consciousness means that no matter how objective we may strive to be, we will never be able to perceive anyone, or anything for that matter, without simultaneously perceiving ourselves. Ultimately this is because individuated consciousness is something of a trick. Although the analogy is flawed dimensionally, we can liken our perception of self and therefore other to a string that has been folded back on itself. When traced back to its source, Life, self becomes revealed as other, and vice versa.

In practical terms, what this means for us is that interpersonal relationship can be very slippery ground. By changing our sense of self, we change our relationships with others automatically—even to the point that we may believe that the other is the one who has changed. What this also means is that what we perceive as the shortcomings or faults of others are in reality reflections in some sense of our wounding. Our dislike of someone's impatience, for example, is itself a form of impatience, just as our judgment of someone's lifestyle reflects to some degree the threat or challenge we perceive that person's lifestyle makes on our own, revealing doubts or fears about how we ourselves live.

This kind of mirroring, or projection, is a common, natural part of our everyday world. It is important to recognize, therefore, that when in our relations with others we bump up against things that bring up strong negative emotional reactions in us that we have in effect rubbed up against some of our own wounding. It's as if we need projection to become aware of aspects of our wounding that are out of conscious awareness. And if there's a negative response within us, it can only because we are in some way expressing or holding similar or related vibrations. Otherwise we wouldn't have a negative reaction. It's like this knock-knock joke:

"Knock, knock."

"Who's there?"

"Always."

"Always who?"

"It's always you."

If someone triggers us, it can only be because there is something to be triggered.

From the perspective that trusts Life to guide and shape us our highest experiences and expressions of love, this way that we have of seeing our own wounding through our interactions with others, in other words emotional triggering, is a very good thing. When we recognize that others can not make us feel anything, that what we feel is in essence who we are and therefore our own responsibility, being triggered becomes an opportunity for emotional healing. Of course it may not feel so great, especially when we unconsciously react defensively and therefore offer resistance to our emotional healing, but once we have learned to respond with recognition for what is actually happening, we find liberation rather than constriction and anxiety.

Without this basic understanding, without the basic trust that Life is bringing to us exactly what we need to heal and grow, we will most likely become locked in various loops of victim consciousness. Victim consciousness is the false ego outlook that has our heels dug in for full-out resistance to our experience as an attempt to control Life. In victim consciousness we feel we are being tormented by others and by Life, and we steel ourselves in defensiveness. The end result of such resistance to experience is first of all insensitivity; we become desensitized to feeling.

Next comes armoring; we plate our bodies, attitudes and behaviors with defensiveness, a virtual array of attacking, withdrawing and delusional camouflaging. In the end of course, since Life relentlessly works to open our hearts, we will invite true, perhaps devastating crisis into our lives because only such force can break through our armoring to touch our hearts. This is the ultimate irony: we steel ourselves against love, which is what we most desire.

Currently in our culture we are largely armored to the teeth. It is not yet a part of our collective understanding that universal love in the forms of gratitude, worthiness, praise, compassion and trust is the guiding truth of our authentic being. We don't yet recognize that emotion is the force of our evolution as beings of love, and we certainly are not yet clear about the nature and purpose of emotional triggering and projection. Eventually, however, we will get it, and humanity will make an evolutionary leap beyond current expectations.

In the meanwhile, we must continue to heal and grow, and there is no more potent way to do this than to create conscious, unconditional relationships with those we love. Such relationships are built on the understanding of our divine natures and unconditional worthiness. The truth of every moment, in other words, is love, and we can make choices in our relationships to reflect that truth. To change the patterns and beliefs of our culture we must work through and heal the wounding inherited from our families, and then apply our new, conscious relationships to the task of accepting and applying in the world our true power, which is the power of universal love.

Of course we have to recognize that healing the inherited wounds of our families through conscious relationship requires a kind of relating that was generally not modeled to us in our own families, and the relating of conscious relationship also goes far beyond the kinds of relationships we typically find on television or at the movie theater. As stated earlier, we first of all need to trust in the very design and intention of Life to indeed guide and shape us to our greatest potentials. We also need to learn and continue to learn to trust and follow our hearts, to do and say that which we feel will create greater love in our lives—however unpopular those urgings may be. And since we must accept the truth of our emotional woundedness, we need to practice discernment, which in relationship develops largely out of heartfelt, honest communication.

Fear of Intimacy

Resistance to such trust, heart and open communication is due primarily to our fear of true intimacy. We can never heal our primary wounds unless we agree to touch them, bring them out into the open and light where they can be revealed for how they distort our self's sense of worth and purpose, but we resist. We resist because at the core of our conditional ego or false self we fear that we will be rejected, that we will not get the love we know we need. So we hold back from stepping into the unknown, into the part of us that is ironically beyond fear and where we are authentically unconditional.

What many people mean when they say that they desire intimacy is that they desire for someone to meet their core emotional needs for safety, nurturance and guidance. But that is not true intimacy. It is not true intimacy when you want someone else to deeply approve of you and acknowledge you or even take care of you. Those are great things and wonderful to experience, but they stop short of true intimacy. Having very specific ideas of what another person should be like or should do before you will open your heart to that person is not the path to intimacy but the path to control. If you are so clear about what you desire for someone else to do or be, then what you are looking for is your self, not intimacy. Your formula for love in such a case is conditional, and you will probably find disappointment after disappointment until you finally understand that your fear is controlling your desire for what you thought was true love.

Intimacy in relationship means stepping into the unknown. It is a step of trust to go beyond fear and the false self to where unparalleled healing and love can fill and inspire us. In intimacy we drop the defenses, and let come what may come. This requires trust and faith because we must know first in our hearts and minds that we can not ever really be hurt, that all we ever protect and defend is the woundedness of our false self. Unconditional is exactly that, unconditional. The need we feel we have for the perfect partner or the perfect circumstances is in the end nothing more than our fear, the defense of our woundedness.

The truth is that however ready we are for true intimacy is a measure of how well we love ourselves. In other words, the more we have healed our core woundedness and are free from regret and resentment, the more we will be available for unconditional, intimate relationship with those we love. Others, it must be repeated, do not hurt us emotionally. Our emotional pain is the conflict between our conditional identity and the truth of our authentic, unconditional being. In truth there is never anything to regret, nor anyone or anything to resent, and such emotions in our relationships are signs of our own wounding keeping us from the gift of true intimacy.

That we attract people into our lives who have the unerring ability to reflect our wounding back to us is part of the beauty of Life's system for healing us and leading us to our divine potential. Our difficulty is that we generally do not recognize or understand what is going on, and this is due to the fact that the depth of our wounding has not been adequately explained to us. Culturally, in fact, we are for the most part emotionally clueless.

Life, however, makes up in part for our cluelessness by making sure that we seek out that which will highlight our wounding. In one sense this might be seen as something of a dirty trick, but it also confirms Life's relentlessness regarding our healing. So we blithely project our core needs onto others, only to be disappointed when they of course can't truly meet them—at least not how we want them to. We also have the uncanny ability of reliving and recreating the dysfunctional patterns of our upbringing or even of our parents' upbringing, again so that they may be healed and tran-scended.

Once we become aware of the dynamics of mirroring, much of our lives starts to make more sense. Life is never interested in hiding our wounding from us, so often it is right there out in the open to see, as long as we know what to look for. For the more difficult or stuck areas of our wounding, we would be wise to look at the model-ing that informed the creation of our identity. As has been repeatedly proven, in terms of our beliefs and attitudes, words do not count nearly as much as modeled behavior. A parent who smokes, for ex-ample, will never find the words to balance out the statement being modeled that smoking is not only okay, it's the choice of the child's idealized parent.

Children not only learn to walk and talk in manners quite simi-lar to their parents, they also unknowingly take on the unspoken beliefs that are reflected in the actions or non-actions of the par-ents. In this way many assumptions about Life and one's value or worthiness are passed from one generation to the next without a word ever being spoken, and these assumptions are often supporting the wounding that seems most difficult for us to see and get at. This chapter's exercise for experiential understanding can be adapted for helping to identify the unconscious modeling that has gone on in your family and society regarding the core emotional needs we all have for safety, nurturance and guidance.

In the final chapter we will take a closer look at modeling, espe-cially for how it relates to our views of work and creativity. It is also time for us to define emotional enlightenment and its relationship to emotional maturity, as well as consider the nature of work in the creation of the authentic self.

Chapter Four Main Points

1. True self-discovery means recognizing that the source of our magical creation is within us. Practical Application: This understanding empowers us to be more consciously involved in the creation of our lives and to see that we are in a very real sense the source of our own suffering.

2. Giving up control means accepting that Life will offer us exactly what we need at all times to shape and guide us to our greatest potentials. Practical Application: When we understand that our desire to control our lives is greatly influenced by our wounding, we learn to work more harmoniously with Life's efforts to guide us.

3. Our emotional wounding does not define our identity but is the energy we can use to fuel our transcendence. Practical Application: When we cease to see our wounding as negative we can use it to inspire our growth and create the authentic self.

4. The proof of our core wounding is in our struggling and our suffering. Practical Application: Knowing that our false ego is the source of our struggling and suffering teaches us to go deeper into our being for healing.

5. True emotional healing can begin when we recognize that on the most fundamental level of our identity we have been had—what we've thought about ourselves and the world is simply wrong. Practical Application: When we have the experience of this kind of genuine self-discovery we also realize that it is everyone's story, and this opens our capacity for compassion.

6. Whatever stories we have about ourselves and Life, our emotional wounding will be woven into their very fabric. Practical Application: Recognizing the self-fulfilling nature of core beliefs serves to expose how we create our lives in part to reveal our woundedness.

7. We are evolutionarily designed to transcend the three patterns of defensive reaction (attack, desensitize, withdraw). Practical Application: Knowing these patterns helps us to identify them in our behaviors so that we may grow beyond them.

8. Mindful sensory experience is the way to gracefully resolve emotional distress. Practical Application: We can learn to transcend defensiveness and heal our emotional wounding through the practice of mindful sensory experience.

9. The core emotional needs for safety, nurturance and guidance are involved in our journey from emotional dependence to emotional maturity. Practical Application: When we learn to look for these emotional needs in our relationships with others and with ourselves we are better able to create unconditional or win/win relationships.

10. To take advantage of relationship mirroring for emotional healing we need to clearly understand emotional triggering, projection, and familial modeling. Practical Application: When we understand that we will never be able to perceive anyone without simultaneously perceiving ourselves we begin to appreciate the basic interconnectedness of everyone—which makes conscious, unconditional relationship easier and more desirable. Moreover, when we understand that attracting people into our lives to mirror our wounding back to us is part of Life's system for healing us and leading us to our potential we can heal more quickly and gracefully.

Exercise for Experiential Understanding

This exercise provides a way to practice mindful sensory experience as well as a method for amplifying the energies of unconditional love that are already a part of your being. You will need a quiet place and at least twenty minutes of uninterrupted solitude. A variation involving the core emotional needs will be given at the end.

Universal love is what makes sense of all emotions, and acts like true north for our emotional evolution and personal growth. As such, it is a complex energetic, composed and woven of unconditional energies in whose synergy we are guided and enriched as we grow into ever greater understanding and experience of the universal love that creates and supports our being. This meditation exercise will help you sort out and compose the many strands of universal love that are the foundation of your identity so that you may fulfill your potentials for creativity and true, unconditional intimacy with others.

Find a place to sit comfortably, either in meditation pose or on a chair with a straight back. If you are sitting in a chair, make sure your feet can be placed squarely on the floor. Place your hands on your knees, palms up, and put your fingers in the given positions. At all times maintain a freely flowing breath. For each step of the Universal Love Meditation say the word (such as Gratitude) either silently to yourself or out loud, and then simply pay attention to what you feel and think in response. From time to time you may wish to repeat the word. Pay attention only; this is a practice in mindfulness. Later if you wish you can try to make more sense of your experiences. Allow 3 to 5 minutes for each step. (You may wish to record the following, perhaps substituting "I" for "you," on a tape recorder, then play it back and follow the instructions you have given yourself. Be sure to allow several minutes for silence between the steps.)

1. Gratitude (thumbs and pinkie fingers touching)

Gratitude is appreciation and thankfulness for all that affirms and supports us. Connect with whatever gratitude you feel (or don't feel) at the moment, whether for family, friends, love, health—just allow whatever it is to bubble up into your consciousness. Feel it in your body, and let all the forms of gratitude you are feeling to be expressed inwardly.

2. Worthiness (thumbs and ring fingers touching)

Worthiness refers to the truth that we are already absolutely worthy, and that our living this truth comes from embracing the path that is shaping us to our highest expression. Connect with your own worthiness. For now, focus on your worthiness, even though it is true that all are worthy. Feel into your self image, and what it is you like and dislike about yourself. Connect with how it feels in your body. As best you can, touch in with your ultimate Divinity, your essential Being that is completely worthy, completely Love. Remember also that your worthiness is based on that Love. You are completely worthy simply because you love, and because you open yourself to being loved.

3. Praise (thumbs and middle fingers touching)

Praise for the joyous creative force of all life, including your own. Praise is a generosity of spirit, a creative expression of the Love that is you. You praise life with your love of live, whether in your relationships (as a friend, lover, father, mother, sister, brother), or simply in your words and feelings of praise to the All-Loving All. You praise life with your creativity, either as a creative artist, or at work, or even when you find a clever way to do something in a new way. Self-care is an especially potent form of praise, for it demonstrates your gratitude for life, and your worthiness. When you are Love, every breath, every thought, every action is praise. Giving love and receiving love are both forms of praise.

4. Compassion (thumbs and pointer fingers touching)

Compassion maintains the integrity of self and asks for nothing. It is the recognition that everyone is unconditionally divine and struggling to know and express that truth. Connect with your feel-ings of compassion for others, for all Beings. Genuine, authentic compassion arises from the understanding that we are all struggling, either consciously or unconsciously, with the same problem: how to know ourselves as Love Itself. Everyone we meet or see is involved in this process, this same journey. Devotional Compassion, the deep-est form of compassion, arises with the experience that we all share the same Heart.

5. Trust (hands together with the compassion thumb/finger positions maintained)

Trust grows from experiencing the truth that you will be met with guidance and support for each step you take to live your au-thentic life. Tune into how well you trust the truth that Life is relentlessly working with you to guide and shape you to your highest potentials for creativity and Love. Whatever steps you take toward acting on that truth are met with grace, with what you need in the moment for you to realize yourself as an expression of the All-Lov-ing All, indeed as Love Itself. Trust comes from the understanding that whatever is in your life, whether or not it feels good, is there to facilitate your evolution. Understanding and experiencing that this is true, that Life works in concert with our efforts to reach our po-tentials for genius, for expressing the Love of the One Heart, brings us back to Gratitude, completing the circle.

Closing: Place your hands in praye position at your heart center (sternum). Or, keeping your hands in the trust position, bring your hands overhead, then slowly bring them down the front of your body as far as you can. Then, bring them to rest at prayer position.

Core Needs Variation

It is also possible to do a similar meditation to gain greater understanding for how your core needs for safety, nurturance and guidance have been met and are currently being met. Instead of using the hand positions for the unconditional love ladder, place your hands in prayer position either resting on your lap or held up against your chest. Next, one at a time say the word for each of the core needs, either silently or aloud, and pay attention to what you feel and imagine. Stay with each need for about 5 minutes. As in the universal love meditation, this is an exercise in mindful sensory experience, so refrain from a lot of analysis and interpretation until you are completely finished.

Questions for Contemplation

How have I been had? Where along the way on my journey have I been deceived, betrayed or tricked? And how have those experiences been teachers for me? How do I feel about the idea that all of those experiences were reflections of the greatest betrayal of all—the betrayal of my Self?

Notes:

Enlightened Creative Expression

So, is our emotional healing ever done? Can we ever unwind our core wounding to the point that it is completely gone, or at least virtually non-existent? The answer from our wisdom traditions indicates that yes, it is possible and has been done. Permanent freedom from self-judgment and emotional suffering has been reported from virtually all wisdom traditions, including of course Christianity and Buddhism. Moreover, it is always reported that such a way of being in the world is possible for everyone, not just extraordinary women and men.

Such prospects of emotional enlightenment, however, raise important questions. Why can't we find happiness now, today? Do we have to wait for emotional enlightenment just to be happy? And if emotional enlightenment is as rare as it seems to be, what are *my* chances?

Although Life is clearly far too much to fully wrap our minds around, we can propose some answers to such questions from within the bounds of the understandings already covered. And these answers are both promising and inspiring. Let's start with three foundational understandings already discussed:

1. Life is benign, supporting us to reach our highest potentials for love and creative expression.

2. Transcendence is the nature Life, and therefore of personal growth.

3. Mystery is at the center of our identity.

These three understandings are the touchstones or guideposts of our emotional journeys as we evolve from the dependence of the false ego through to emotional maturity, and then on toward emotional enlightenment. (In other words, the journey from self-discovery on to emotional healing and the creation of the authentic self.) And each leg of the journey brings its own forms of happiness, its own adventures. Yet that happiness will not be realized, our lives not joyous, unless we fully grasp the most amazing thing of all: We are Life, in all its glory. And this journey we are on is the adventure of our waking up to that seemingly impossible, wondrous truth.

The more we can experience the reality of this, the greater will be our happiness, regardless of where we are on the journey. We don't have to wait for emotional enlightenment to be happy. We can be happy today. And the best way to realize our happiness, our joy, on each and every day of this incredible journey is to align ourselves with the truth of our divine identity. There is no end station, no final enlightenment. We are on an infinite journey of greater and greater consciousness and awareness of our identity as Life itself. To know this and experience this is to be delighted, free from the lies and restraints of the false ego. This is the way of love, of knowing ourselves as Life's Lover, and Life's Beloved.

For another way to understand how life-changing this information about our authentic identity can be, consider the layering of choice, desire and identity. Our choices are based directly on our desires, and these desires (whether conscious or unconscious) are based directly on the identity we have accepted for ourselves. Simply uncover the identity associated with the desire, and we will find the leverage point for real change in our lives. Conversely, if we know ourselves to be divine forms or expressions of Life (Life itself, in other words), this will affect our desires, leading to choices in alignment with that authentic identity.

Of course the simple or false ego can be very convincing, which is why it's necessary to understand emotional development and the dynamics of emotional evolution. Throughout the healing process, we must also hold emotional maturity as our goal. Emotional maturity, as we've learned, happens when we take full responsibility for making sure that our primary needs of safety, nurturance and guidance are met in ways that are supportive (win/win) for all. This may be a high standard to reach for and truly meet, but our conscious steps toward emotional maturity will unfailingly be met by the kinds of growth we need to find even greater happiness and creative satisfaction. Remember, Life is benign, transcendence is our nature, and mystery, or the unknown, is at the core of who we are.

Radical Self-Acceptance

In the simplest of terms, there is really only one path out of the darkness and suffering of the conditional ego and false self. This is the road of radical self-acceptance, of fully embracing the truth of our ultimate identity as Life.

The first understanding or step on this yellow brick road is that whatever our experience is at any moment, it is directly reflective of who we are, and is the product of our own perception. With this in mind, we must learn to recognize our wounding and make choices to create the conditions for expressing our true nature. We must, in other words, nurture and develop our own genius. As Life, we are creative geniuses. Look around at nature, and know that this is true. Enjoy and appreciate the creative work of any artist you admire, and know that such genius is also who you are. Life provides us with never-ending opportunities to develop and celebrate our divine creativity, but we must first know that this is indeed who we are before we can really shine.

Becoming responsible for our own authentic well being, the happy radiance of genius, ensures that we learn to face down the lies of the false or conditional self. This is easy of course when things are going well, but at the first sign of a bumpy ride we must accept the reality that our own wounding is responsible for our reactions to our experience. We will also no doubt begin to understand that the identity we hold in our mind may be much different than the identity we embrace at our emotional core. Knowing this, Life continually asks us one question: Who are You? When we consistently respond in ways that reflect the true nature of our divinity, we will know greater and greater love, and greater and greater creativity.

Ultimately it is probably our concern for others that teaches us to take the next step of radical self-acceptance, which is absolute self-approval. Just like Dorothy and her friends in the *Wizard of Oz*, when we love and care for others we are inspired to step out of our own woundedness, and we are then more able to find approval of ourselves from within because we get in touch with the love that we are. Self-approval, however, will eventually bump into the limits imposed by our core woundedness, and we will have to learn the lesson that we can love others and be loved only to the degree of our own self-love. Any self-negation or unworthiness we hold in our hearts will put limits on how much we can love and be loved.

The third step of radical self-acceptance is self-acknowledgment. Like Dorothy's Tin Man, Scarecrow and Cowardly Lion, we need recognition, but our recognition will have to come from within if we hope to ever break free of our self-limiting false self. Our choices to take care of our bodies, to engage only in unconditional relationship with others, and to be open to and accepting of Life's guiding hand must come from our desire to honor and acknowledge ourselves for our innate goodness and worthiness. Truly taking care of ourselves is the best way we can demonstrate our self-love to ourselves, and this kind of self-acknowledgment will empower us to take further steps in our healing.

At some point, our radical self-acceptance will mature into genuine emotional maturity, and we will know greater satisfaction with our lives than ever, and we will also have periods of great creativity. From there, the seeds of emotional enlightenment have been sown, and we will come to know great emotional wisdom. In essence, emotional enlightenment is the experience of living when you know that you are the Beloved. You have transcended infantile neediness and have the experiential understanding that love surrounds you, that grasping for it will only bring suffering because that grasping is done out of a sense of lack, which is untrue. And in the end it is only untruth that bring suffering.

When emotionally enlightened, there are no attachment dramas—as Lover and the Beloved there is an intrinsic wholeness to your being. Of course there will still be change, and further evolution, but you will be free of the sufferings of longing for the Beloved—either in yourself or in another. Knowing that you are Life, you love and accept love without shame, guilt or hesitation. You experience delight at Life's incredible display.

Emotional enlightenment can be compared to when Dorothy looks behind the curtain to find the bumbling wizard, but with a very significant difference. This time when you look behind the curtain you find your Self, and the fiction that is your defended ego becomes totally revealed. In fact, as the Lover/Beloved (the realized transcendent ego), there is no separate you to speak of. This affords you tremendous freedom, for you are now released from attachment dramas, which are based on your seeking, and on your sense of some kind of lack. Simultaneously, your body and your imagination make great leaps, as they are one with your emotional self. Physical vitality and creative artistry literally soar.

Equally important is the new vision that you acquire. No longer involved in the push-me pull-you of emotional entanglement with others, you can see much more clearly how conflict at all levels (the personal, the social, the political, the transpersonal) is the result of emotional immaturity and the seeking of control. With emotional enlightenment comes the fruit of devotional compassion, which is grounded in the experiential understanding that we all share the same Heart.

The Love Law of Manifestation

As incredible as emotional enlightenment is, we do not need emotional enlightenment to be happy—genuinely, positively happy and full of joy and delight. That is available to us every day, no matter where we are on our journey. One way to experience this is to practice the love law of manifestation. As you are no doubt aware, there are a lot of manifestation practices and rituals available these days, most based on the premise that we can have whatever we want. In fact, the universe is apparently wired to give us what we want, without fail. "Ask and you shall receive," Jesus is reported to have said, for example. The hitch seems to be that either we don't know what we want, or we have unconscious programming or self-sabotaging mechanisms that keep us from getting what we want. And so we run around trying to undo the programming or trying to get in touch with the self-sabotage—-which is always about confusions we have about our identity so it's great to be aware of such things.

But there is a much simpler reason for why we don't get what we try and manifest, whether it's the new car or the new darling. These things or people or opportunities are not what we want. If we think that we want the Mercedes or the house in the mountains, we are to some degree deluding ourselves. To rewrite The Beatles: all we want is love. We want the *feeling* that we imagine the Benz will give us, or that we imagine the soul mate or the chateau will provide.

This makes the whole story of Life in one sense delightfully simple. Because the universe is indeed wired to give us what we want, and all we want is love, we are truly talking of a match made in heaven. And it gets even better. Rather than making a list of what we love, or cutting pictures out of a magazine, the way to manifest what we want (love) is simply to consciously love and appreciate whatever is in our lives right now that we already love and appreciate. This will increase the love vibe around us, immediately attracting more love.

This is the Love Law of Manifestation: Love Loves Love. And since Life unfailingly guides and shapes us to our greatest potentials for love, by really loving what you already love you will be attracting exactly what you need for your continued growth in love—not just what you think you need. In short, if we make it a practice to truly love whatever it is that we already love, our lives will be increasingly filled with what we love—and with what loves us. There is no more beautiful way to live.

This also means that whenever we desire something new, we can take this as a sign that we are ready for greater love. So in addition to loving and appreciating what is already in our lives, we can begin to make room for this even greater love to come into our lives by looking and feeling in beyond the form of our new desire. For example, if we wish to have a bigger house (remember from Dorothy that a house is psychological symbol for identity), we can focus in on the feeling of that new, bigger house. This is done perhaps best during meditation, or any time when we can slow our breath and calm the mind.

When the form of our desire gives way to the feelings aroused by our imagining, we have found the essence of our new desire. In this example, it may actually be a desire for a greater sense of community that lies at the heart of a desire for a bigger house, such as more space for gatherings and guests. Feel into that desire for the greater love of community until you can feel it throughout your body. Allow it and embrace it. This is your acceptance of the greater love being offered by your desire. The form that this greater love takes in your life may or may not be the bigger house, but it will certainly arrive. And why not? You are Life's Beloved, and you will be continuously invited to greater and greater experiences of love.

And what of envy, greed and revenge—or other such desires we may feel? These too are indications that we are ready for greater love in our lives. If for example we desire the bigger house in order to outdo our brother or sister or to show our parents how wrong they were about us, then our desire is based on inner feelings of lack. By getting in touch with and deeply feeling in our body those inner feelings of have been bested, cheated or wronged, we open the door to healing, and to the generosity of love that supports and encourages all to flourish. We can also be certain that the manifested form of what we desire will be perfectly suited to our unique journey to greater love.

The Work of Creation

Once we have managed to become emotionally mature through the practice of radical self-acceptance, our work in the world will naturally take on new meaning, and be more of an adventure we look forward to than a task we would rather not do. This then, the creative expression of the authentic self *in the world*, is what follows self-discovery and emotional healing, and must be the next subject for our attention.

Perhaps no word cuts as quickly to the heart of how we feel about ourselves and our lives than "work." Work is the expression of ourselves in the world, and therefore to a large degree seems to define our life's meaning and purpose. Work in this sense refers then to much more than one's job or employment, and it encompasses unpaid work like parenting and studying. Work, put simply, is our creative expression; and in psycho-emotional terms it is the daily activity that creates our sense of self.

Seeing work in this way reveals how work reflects our emotional development, and why meaningful creative work is the natural progression from self-discovery and emotional healing. First we discover that we are not who we thought we were, but that like Dorothy in the *Wizard of Oz* we are much more powerful, capable and beautiful than we had ever imagined. Next comes our emotional healing, where we transform our core wounding into our authentic self, our true way of being in the world. It is in fact during the time of our emotional healing that follows genuine self-discovery that we create our authentic self—and it is perhaps even the first sense we have of our life's true work.

That each of us has a true work, a calling or destiny, is an idea that shows up again and again in our wisdom traditions, yet it appears clear from our actions as a society that we really don't believe it. Certainly we believe in callings in general, and we talk and tell stories about those folks who have had callings and found success, but the idea that each human being has a calling or true work that awaits being awakened and brought into being is not something that we take to heart. If we did, our parenting practices and education systems would be quite different—as would our society as a whole.

The truth of the matter is that the false self and our emotional wounding is what keeps us from knowing and acting on our calling, our genius. That urge that each person feels to be free, to be liberated from so much suffering and struggle is the call, but for the most part we either don't know how seriously we should take it or don't feel that it is real. After all, when we look around, what we see is that suffering is the expected way of adulthood. Adults even do their best to shield children from finding out what's in store for them later on, and we bemoan the plight of those whom we feel have missed out on the relatively carefree world of childhood.

This romanticized notion of childhood comes out of our own despair. We sacrifice and suffer nobly, but for the most part we have given up on the urgings and callings we once had to be free. Somewhere along the way we became resigned to our adult fates and were encouraged and pressured to give up on such pipe dreams and to start wishing parts of our days away like everyone else. Such frustration and ignorance regarding our true potential influences us to ignore any calls for liberation, or at best to treat them as something perhaps possible for our children if we can provide them with the advantages we never had.

Of course we can never give anyone such freedom, not even our children. We can help prepare the soil for the transcendence of others, but in the end it is up to each of us to accept our own worthiness and step through the gate of self-discovery. And in the end this is probably the best we can do for others, especially our children. The more that we are able to stand in the truth of our being, the more we will create a world that can heal and transcend its own woundedness. Not only will our example inspire others, but our authentic actions, our work, will create increasingly greater options for others to use for support and guidance. And if we are parents, we will break many of the cycles of woundedness that are passed from generation to generation, creating a legacy potentially much more valuable than any fruits of economic security.

And for those who do consciously choose the path of self-discovery and healing, once we feel our divine essence and the potential of our authentic being, we will start to become aware or more greatly aware of our calling. The emotional healing we then do to free ourselves from our conditional ego creates more and more the authentic being that is who we truly are. Moreover, the natural expressions of our talents, and the surfacing of unknown and unrealized capabilities and potentials, inspires our creative or true work. It is as if each of us is in fact a seed, and we must somehow break through the shell of ourselves to discover what kind of being, what kind of genius, we are destined to become.

Seen in this way, our false self is rightly viewed not as something bad, but as a stage in our growth. The problem is that we are a world of seeds, so when we look around we misunderstand. We think: to be human is to be a seed, and being a seed means a lot of struggle and suffering. And we think: I'll be strong like everyone else to earn respect and approval for my suffering because that's the best thing available. And as we near the end of our lives we think: I've done the best I could and I'm proud of my life for the most part, so let me die without any more suffering.

Our pride is honorable, but it is misplaced. Life tries to shake us out of our shells, our seed casings, and as much as we desire to be free of so much struggle, we hold our seed shells as close as possible with the idea that we have to protect ourselves. But we are mistaken. We must break out of our seed mentality, our seed culture, if we genuinely desire to find out who we are and to reach our potentials for love and creativity. As a society we are stuck in pre-self-discovery, unaware of our truth, our beauty, and our grandeur. And for the most part, our fear of letting Life work through us to awaken our potential means that we do our best to create a world where being closed-up and resisting our greatness is the norm.

Resistance, however, means more struggling and suffering, because what we are resisting is our own evolution. Occasionally the pressure to transcend becomes more than we can bear and we break open for a while, but before long we've found our way into a new shell with maybe a little more room. In a world of seeds, it feels scary to go beyond and become a free and liberated being.

Eventually we won't have a choice. As it currently stands, our collective resistance to our emotional and therefore spiritual evolution is creating even more pressure for us to transcend our ways. We're of course doing it to ourselves, and as always we have choices to make that could make our journey more graceful. We even know that we're making things increasingly worse for ourselves by our lifestyles and how we treat our planet—and sometimes we even see how our conception of our planet as an "other" (as if we were somehow not interdependent with the planet) is crazy talk. But our heels are dug in deep.

At this rather desperate or despairing stage of humanity's ignorance of itself in light of the clear evidence of how we are destroying our world and therefore ourselves, it's useful to start imagining how our emotional evolution will alter our perception of work and therefore the insanity of our economy's values. It's useful because in the end we will dream our way out of our problems, out of our shells and our denial, and the sooner we all begin to do that the better things will go. So from the perspective of emotional development, we must start imagining a world where true work, inspired by callings, becomes the norm. In other words, we will know we are well on our way to creating an authentic world, a world not of seeds but of authentic beings, when human potential is revered as our greatest resource.

When work is seen and practiced as the art of creation, as our conscious contribution to the joy of living that is the source of Life's sense- and dream-making, then we will be living according to our true potentials. In such a world the creative expression of the authentic self will be the focus of our doing, and this will necessarily include respect for the earth, simple abundance, and lifelong learning. It will be a beautiful world where we will still have our problems, but we will understand that these problems have their source within us, and we will respond accordingly and as wisely as we know how.

But what about today? Can't we as individuals already begin creating and inhabiting such a world? As soon as we accept that our problems are within us, that we live according to the fearful conditioning of our false self, we begin to create this world for ourselves. It is already possible to live in an authentic world because the truth of our authentic being is available to us in each moment. Radical self-acceptance is the first step of self-discovery, as we have already seen. And in the healing that follows, we create a world for ourselves that reflects our growing acceptance of the truth of who we truly are.

There is, in other words, a direct link between our emotional evolution and our creative expression or our true work. As we heal our core wounding we emerge as emotionally mature individuals able to recognize and actualize our highest creative expression. Specifically, in terms of our creative work, this involves three insights:

1.   Understanding that wherever you are *now* is perfect for your calling;

2.   Recognizing how your parental modeling about work and creativity influences how well you are able to hear and heed your calling;

3.   Recognizing how the societal and institutional modeling that shapes your ideas of what is acceptable or possible also strongly influences how well you are able to create your true work in the world.

1. Now is Perfect

It is never too late to do your true work. Wherever you are in your life, all your experiences have led to and prepared you for doing your Great Work—no experience, no single thought even, has ever been out of place or wasted. In fact, from the point of view of your calling, your Great Work, you have never made one single mistake. Your choices, and the consequences of those choices, have perfectly shaped and prepared you to find and express the love and talents of your authentic being.

How can this be so? How can it be that no matter what our experiences have been, no matter what our age or personal circumstances, that every moment has been perfect for leading us to our true work? The reason is that a person's Great Work is a natural expression of that person's authentic being, which includes *all* of her or his experiences. Authentic being is only possible when there is unconditional self-acceptance and self-approval. From the point of view of authentic being, our past mistakes and our past accomplishments are equally valid for having created the present moment where we recognize and acknowledge our absolute worthiness.

True work is the natural creative expression of the authentic self, which means that our highest creative potential is reached through the path of self-discovery and healing. And since work is the activity that creates our sense of self, our evolving transcendent self will necessarily include and integrate all of our experiences. Ultimately we will understand how even those unconscious choices rooted in our wounding have been creating the conditions for us to recognize and engage in our true work. This is because the conditions of our lives, including the wounding we inherited from our families and culture, are ideally suited for creating the opportunities for us to grow out of our seed-being to become the unique expression of divine consciousness that is our potential.

To say such a thing implies that each of us has a kind of destiny or fate that awaits in potential for us to recognize and activate, and this is true insofar as we also accept that this destiny or fate finds a form of our own making. Once we step outside the confines of the conditional self, we will create our authentic being starting from and out of whatever our experiences have been to that point. Our potential destiny or Great Work is not highly specified, in other words, but is the energy for a way of being from which we can create a unique, authentic self.

This differs from standard ways of viewing destiny or fate because it does not imply predestination of any sort. Yes, when we begin to live authentically we will be presented with opportunities that are so perfect that they may seem to have been predestined, but this is simply how Life steps forth to help us when we are making choices that are in harmony with our deepest truths. To mistake such opportunities for the hand of Fate is to invite being blind-sided by the consequences of choices rooted in our remaining unconscious wounding.

Differentiating the path of our highest potential from ideas of fate or destiny that are linked to predestination actually serves to emphasize that engaging in our true work can begin at any time in our lives. It is always possible for us to tap into the potential energies of our authentic being, and to begin creating a world for ourselves based on our highest truths. To do so we should first of all recognize the forces that shaped and continue to maintain our conditional self so that we can identify the unconscious decisions we make that keep us from going forward.

What this means of course is that at the root of all of our ideas about Life and work is our emotional woundedness. Learning to recognize and understand this woundedness, together with realizing that it can be gracefully healed, is truly the art of emotional wisdom. The ability to reach our highest potentials for love and creativity, which are the foundation of true work, is gained through the processes of self-discovery and emotional healing. It is the journey we were born for, and it begins whenever we can accept that it can begin with every moment.

2. Parental Modeling

As much importance as we give to words, we also know that they are not nearly as powerful as our actions. This turns out to be especially true for all of the values and ideas about Life that we learn from our parents—including those regarding creativity and work. Long before we ever learn to express ourselves maturely with spoken language, we have been immersed and then continue for many years to be engaged in a world of modeling that unconsciously teaches us most of what we learn from our parents.

Such modeling is extremely powerful. And it can also be very difficult to see. Our folk wisdom teaches us that the apple doesn't fall far from the tree, but what it doesn't explicitly tell us is that self-limiting or even self-destructive modeling is as equally ingrained as the shared speech patterns and mannerisms. Moreover, the actual forms that the modeling takes may be quite different. A parent who smokes, for example, is teaching far more than the obvious lesson that smoking is good. The child may therefore not become a smoker, but may express the modeling through other self-destructive behaviors.

For this reason, it is wise to closely examine as best as possible what modeling we received from our parents around the issues of personal creativity and work. It is certain that all problems or frustrations we have regarding our work in the world will be directly linked in some fashion to the modeling we received at home. This does not mean that our parents are in any real sense to blame for our work and creativity issues. Each of us is responsible for our own self-discovery and healing, and we have in any case personalized the modeling to fit our potentials and temperaments. Becoming aware of the connections between our modeling and our frustrations or difficulties helps us to understand just how we are being guided by Life to break through and tap into our divine potential.

It is also important to recognize the role that our emotional idealization of our parents plays. As discussed in earlier chapters, emotional idealization of our parents is a natural part of our emotional and psychological development. This idealization not only provides a needed sense of security, it also internalizes within us the emotional strengths and emotional wounding of our parents. Such emotional idealization can therefore be a source of self-limitation whenever we refrain from doing what is best for ourselves because of how it may affect our parents' approval of us.

Emotional idealization can also be a problem whenever we are unaware of how the idealization keeps us from seeing the inherited wounding that must be healed. Self-limiting ideas about work and creativity expressed by our parents either in words or through modeling can have extreme effects on the choices we make for ourselves—especially on how well we can hear and heed our calling.

Emotional idealization and parental modeling are two very powerful forces on our psyches that often work hand-in-hand. For this reason, and also in light of all the changes that have recently taken place regarding work and gender, it is wise to recognize and understand how we have been affected by the modeling of our parents. Take out some paper and a pen to write out some answers to these questions. *Creativity* for our purposes here will refer to any expression of self that visibly gives joy to self and others. If you are inspired to follow up on a line of thinking, do so.

- How did your parents express themselves creatively?

- How closely linked were their personal expressions of creativity and their work? (Remember that our definition of work is not necessarily economically based.)

- What were their attitudes, as expressed in their lives and in their words, about the connection between work and creativity?

Once we have taken this very general survey of the modeling we received from our parents, we need to examine our own behaviors and attitudes and look for correlations.

- Is your current work your highest creative expression, or leading you to your highest creative expression?

- If not, can you find connections to the modeling you experienced about creativity and work? (A connection can also be a reaction.)

- What are your beliefs about work and creativity? Do you feel work is a necessary evil, or do you have a different understanding about work?

- Do you look forward to your work? Or do you endure it for what it materially provides you with?

These questions are of course only a start, but they will begin to give you a sense for how much our views on work and creativity are indeed the result of the modeling we experienced at home. Those who have in some way gone against the modeling they grew up with will most likely have a keener sense of the power of modeling in this respect, and those who have more or less followed the modeling of their familial home life will perhaps have a keener sense for how the changes in society have created new twists in work and creativity issues that their parents did not experience. In both cases we can experience firsthand how it is through work and creativity issues that we as individuals most directly interact with society.

3. Societal Modeling

When we take a step back to view societal changes on a broad scale, we can begin to get a general sense for the evolution of work as a function of emotional evolution. As was explored earlier, consciousness is a force intent on self-awareness, and in emotional terms we can now take that one step further to state that consciousness is a force intent on self-discovery. What this means is that being aware that one is aware is only the first step. From there we are faced with an evolutionary pressure to reach emotional maturity, which among other things means knowing and accepting our divine and unconditional worthiness.

On the personal level this is perhaps more readily accepted and understood, but since our society is an extension of our personal lives, the evolutionary pressures will be felt quite strongly as we as individuals evolve beyond the attitudes and forms of work currently sanctioned by society. For example, we are living in a time when our ideas of work are largely limited to specific forms of economic activity, and this economic activity is enmeshed in systems of unmanageable and unsustainable material waste—as well as the poisoning of our air, ground and water. Clearly there will be increasing pressure to overhaul not only our systems that create such waste and pollution but also to transform the very ideas of work that contributed to the creation of our unsustainable and life-threatening systems in the first place.

This evolutionary pressure for change will come in large part from individuals who are evolving emotionally beyond the conditional ego-based systems that underpin our economic systems.

There is, in other words, an institutional and societal consciousness that a society creates, and this consciousness is a reflection in large part of the human forces that created it. A model for doing business or for using energy, for example, functions on the assumptions of those whose behaviors and attitudes made it a working model. This means that the lack of serious concern for emitting poisonous gases into the atmosphere that is such a part of our daily lives says a great deal about our emotional evolution as a society.

Not only does such behavior reveal how little compassion we have for the living organisms of our world (including ourselves!), but it also reveals how far from emotional maturity we are as a society if have not yet learned to meet our individual needs without seriously infringing on the ability of others and other societies to meet theirs. The same could be said for our continued wasteful use of the earth's resources for what we think of as our material needs— but which are in fact emotional needs that we have not learned to maturely meet.

The truth is that we have the knowledge to drastically reduce or eliminate the poisonous emissions into the air, just as we have the knowledge and know-how to do many environmentally-friendly things that we simply do not do. What we must learn is that what we call economic sense (i.e. the waste and pollution of our world) is in fact emotional sense. We do not break out of our unsustainable systems for emotional reasons. We find it convenient to say that such waste and degradation makes economic sense because it shields us from facing the truth of our emotional immaturity. Yes, the modeling of our economic systems is strong, but it is the fact that we are not connected to the experience of our true natures that keeps positive change from occurring.

The same is of course true for the societal modeling that shapes our ideas of what is acceptable or possible in regard to work. In many respects we have entered a new age, the information age, where greater economic value and therefore work value is being placed on information and the exchange of information than ever before. This change signifies the reshaping of our society, as well as the shifting of our forms of work. Yet if we do not evolve emotionally at the same time we will simply overlay the new forms of work with the old emotional wounding.

Changing how we look at work changes how we view ourselves and our relation to our fellow humans. When we begin to see work as the activity that creates our sense of self, we will start to understand the connections between our work issues and our emotional issues. Ideally, our work should allow us to express our creativity in ways that empower us and also contribute to the well being of others. As it currently stands, however, the forms of work that are largely available for us do not allow that. In fact, our work and lifestyle habits create the stresses that decrease our quality of life and lead to chronic and often life-threatening health problems—not to mention our habits for waste and pollution.

Breaking free into new forms of work that do allow us to creatively create ourselves will be made easier by doing the self-discovery and healing work that will evolve us emotionally so that we can tap into the creative energy of our true potential. This is not only the way to greater personal satisfaction, it is also the way for us to evolve as a society.

Back to Kansas

So what's it going to take? How will we ever get to the day when people like their jobs because their jobs are their true work and bring them and others real joy? When will the day come when we do not have to settle for work that is not optimal for our health and well being? How long before we become brave enough to change the destructive ways we measure value in our economies? When will we start educating our young in ways that facilitate rather than hinder their discovery of their divine nature?

The answer is simple and will not change: we will transform our world one person at a time. And we are the ones such creation must start with as we make new choices for ourselves every step of the way.

The work of creation involves recreating the self, day after day. It is a journey of journeys within journeys, and more than anything else it is our emotional experience that provides continuity and de-termines whether we face our daily re-creation with a heavy heart or a sense of hopeful adventure. Unfortunately, many of us feel bur-dened by our lives more than we would care to admit. But it truly doesn't need to be that way. Re-creating the self, or creating the authentic self, or whatever you wish to call the potential for con-tinuous renewal that happens when we tap into the truth of our deepest unconditional reality, is the gateway to a life of genuine sat-isfaction and joy—of true intimacy and true work.

And it all begins with authentic self-discovery. From that time on, nothing will ever be the same because once a seeker has tasted the unconditional self-acceptance of self-discovery there will be no turning back. It is in the fullest sense an initiation into one's true way of being, and as such it marks the beginning of the adventure of becoming truly human.

This profound self-discovery is not the same as initiation into adulthood, though there are strong parallels—which is why *The Wizard of Oz* is often prematurely dismissed as a simple coming-of-age tale. In both kinds of initiations there is a real sense of empowerment, and also a sense of belonging. The differences, how-ever, are telling. In the initiation of self-discovery the empowerment one feels goes beyond the conditional ideas of Life expressed by one's family and society; it is an empowerment of the soul, an awakening to one's identity beyond name, gender and personal history.

The sense of belonging is therefore also different; it is a belonging to one's Self, to all of Life, and it is freedom from the approval brokerings of the conditional self that keep one tied to the expectations and wounding of others. After authentic self-discovery, one recognizes instantly what is self, and what is other, and where lies the responsibility for healing. Moreover, the experience of the Self brings a capacity for forgiveness needed for healing core emotional wounds. And of course, it also brings joy, unquenchable joy at having discovered the incredible truth of Life's love.

Self-discovery. Emotional healing. Creating the authentic self. These are simple words for sacred experiences. Hopefully, the insights and exercises in the pages of this book will be useful for the sacred work of your journey. Best wishes for an exciting adventure of self-discovery, healing, and truly creative work befitting of your genius. And thank you for your contributions toward creating the world of beauty we all know is possible.

Namaste.

Chapter Five Main Points

1.   The three foundational understandings (that Life is benign; transcendence is the nature of Life, and therefore of personal growth; and that mystery is as the center of our identity) are the truths or guideposts of our emotional journeys as we evolve from the dependence of the false ego through to emotional maturity, and then on toward emotional enlightenment. Practical Application: Using these touchstones can provide orientation when we became confused about choices we must make.

2.   We can be happy today, right now. And the best way to realize our happiness, our joy, on each and every day of this incredible journey is to align ourselves with the truth of our divine identity.

Practical Application: When we learn to take responsibility for our own happiness by choosing thoughts and actions that reflect who we really are, we will find the joy and delight we seek.

3. We can love others and therefore only be loved to the degree that we love ourselves. Practical Application: Our desire to honor and acknowledge ourselves will lead us to make choices to take care of our bodies, to engage only in unconditional relationships with others, and to accept Life's guiding hand.

4. Emotional enlightenment is the experience of knowing yourself as Life's Beloved, as well as Life's Lover. Practical Application: Learning to accept and give love equally will bring us closer to being freed of attachment dramas created from a sense of lack.

5. The Love Law of Manifestation explains how Love Loves Love. Practical Application: By getting to the heartfelt feelings of love that are the essence of our desires, we can be clearer about our true desires and allow greater love into our lives.

6. Work is the activity that creates our sense of self. Practical Application: Seeing work in this way reveals how work reflects our emotional development on the path to emotional maturity and emotional enlightenment.

7. Each of us has a true work, a calling or destiny. Practical Application: When we accept this to be true, we can find the courage to do the emotional healing that will reveal our buried calling.

8. Parental modeling about work and creativity influences how well you are able to hear and heed your calling, while societal and institutional modeling influences how well you are able to create your true work in the world. Practical Application: Mapping out the modeling we have received for how it affects how we find and create our true work provides needed insight into why and how we limit or restrict our creative expression so that we may grow.

9. What we call economic sense is in fact emotional sense. Practical Application: When we see work as the activity that creates our sense of self, the connections between our work issues and emotional issues become clearer.

10. Without authentic self-discovery we will never have the capacity for forgiveness that the healing of our core wounding requires. Practical Application: Understanding that we must truly see ourselves and our absolute worthiness in order to heal and create our authentic self is a call to wake up from the hypnotic trance of the conditional self.

Exercise for Experiential Understanding

This exercise is an introductory exercise to help define your highest creative expression. You will need pen and paper.

Step One:

Write down what you would be doing with your life if material needs were not an issue, if for example you had all the money you could ever need. Include in your list as many things that you can imagine, and then order them in terms of importance.

Step Two:

Next make a list of everything you would do with your life if all your needs for emotional nurturance were met. This would mean that you had fulfilling love and companionship in your life, and all the recognition from others that you could ever need. (To make this exercise more effective, exaggerate how honored and respected you are in this fantasy world.)

Step Three:

For this last step, imagine that you have the guidance and support to do anything you want to learn how to do. Assume that you also have your material needs more than adequately met and that you also have your needs for emotional nurturance more than adequately met. Write down everything you would want to learn to do.

Review:

Review your written responses for each step. Does anything strike or surprise you? Go through each step and identify ways in which you could already begin to step forward in these directions. It's not necessary to first of all choose the one thing you should be doing. Instead, watch how Life responds to each of the steps you make to create the dreams you have outlined in these three steps. You may even wish to do this with a friend or a small group, and offer each other emotional support to continue exploring how you could make these or similar dreams come true.

Questions for Contemplation

What one desire have I had in my life for a long time? What daily choices do I make in order to satisfy that one desire? More importantly, can I give a name to the identity out of which this desire springs? Does naming the identity clarify or change the desire? If I stay with the feeling of that desire, what happens in my body? In my mind?

Notes:

INDEX

About the Author

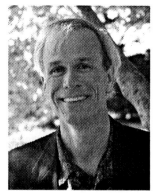

Stephen Bye © 2004

Liam Quirk has lived and traveled extensively throughout the US and Europe, and he currently resides in Bucks County, Pennsylvania. A musician, teacher and nationally certified somatic therapist, Liam has done pioneering work to facilitate our understanding of emotion and human potential. *The Art of Emotional Wisdom* is his first book.

For information on workshops and other events, please visit www.emotionalwisdom.net.

Printed in the United States
40448LVS00007B/61-81

9 781588 321015